AMBROISE PARÉ
Surgeon of the Renaissance

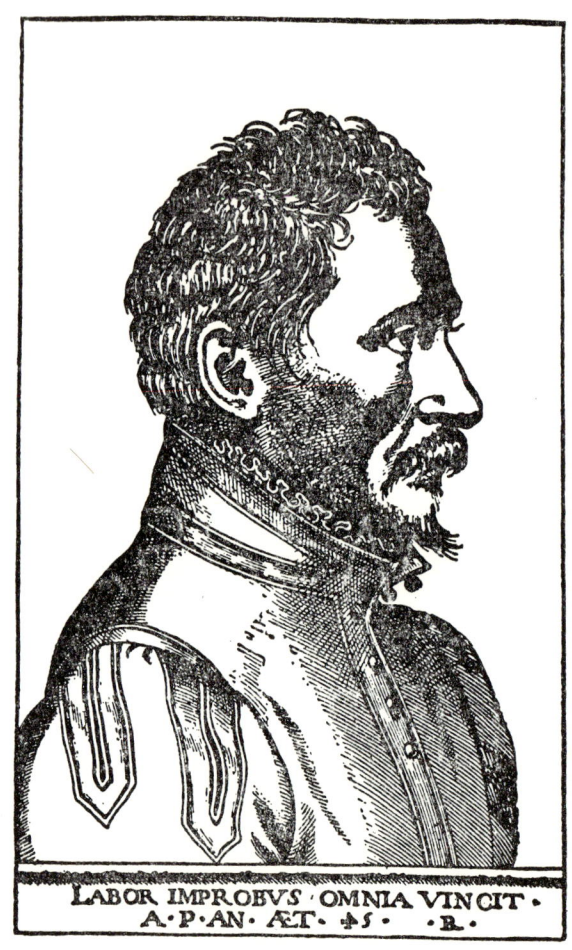

AMBROISE PARÉ, AT THE AGE OF FORTY-FIVE.
(*Anatomie Universelle*, 1561.)

Figure 1. Portrait of Ambroise Paré at the age of forty-five.

AMBROISE PARÉ

Surgeon of the Renaissance

By

WALLACE B. HAMBY, M.D.

*Head, Department of Neurological Surgery
The Cleveland Clinic Foundation
Cleveland, Ohio
Formerly, Professor of Neurological Surgery
University of Buffalo School of Medicine
Buffalo, New York*

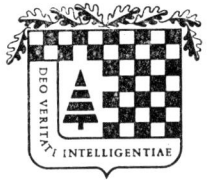

WARREN H. GREEN, INC.
St. Louis, Missouri, U.S.A.

Published by

WARREN H. GREEN, INC.
10 South Brentwood Blvd.
St. Louis, Missouri 63105, U.S.A.

This book is protected
by copyright. No part may
be reproduced in any manner
without written permission
from the publisher.

©1967 by WARREN H. GREEN, INC.
Library of Congress Catalog Card No. 67-19384

WZ
100
P227h
1967

Printed in the United States of America
5-A

To my beloved wife, Mary Jane

Introduction

INTEREST IN Ambroise Paré as a person was revived in 1804, when Napoleon commissioned M. de Lassus to seek out Paré's descendants in Laval, so that they could be honored in the name of their illustrious ancestor. None was found. In 1813, the Bordeaux Society of Medicine staged a prize competition for a eulogy of him. In 1840, J. F. Malgaigne, a French surgeon and later professor of the Faculté de Médecine of Paris, issued a new edition of the old surgeon's *Complete Works*. Going far beyond the specific requirements of his task, Malgaigne made a prodigious search into all aspects of Paré's life. He found several earlier accounts of Paré's life so contradictory as to resemble fiction more than history. Working from original sources as much as possible, he attempted a more accurate presentation. The result was a treasure trove: finally the reader could find, in modern French, almost everything Paré ever wrote and practically everything that was then known of him. Malgaigne's voluminous footnotes resolved many obscure and contradictory ideas of the man and of his works.

Malgaigne's Introduction contained so much personal Paré material that I translated this and it has appeared in English (*Surgery and Ambroise Paré,* University of Oklahoma Press, Norman, Oklahoma, 1965).

In 1887, Dr. Stephen Le Paulmier, a descendant of one of Paré's personal professional enemies, Julien Le Paulmier, added to Malgaigne's store many factual data obtained in a systematic search of historical material available in various French archives, and of which Malgaigne was ignorant. Le Paulmier also found, living near Nemours, one of Paré's descendants who not only had preserved valuable family data, but who also possessed a previously unknown oil painting of Ambroise. Using this source material, Paget and Packard wrote delightful *Lives of Paré,* and they included what to us is his most interesting account, his *Journeys in Divers Places.*

In 1634, Th. Johnson published an English translation of the Latin edition of Paré's Works, the *Opera,* and included a fresh translation of the *Journeys,* that had not been written at the time of the publication of the *Opera.* Johnson's book makes delightful reading, as much for the charm of its 17th century English style as for its contents. This popularity is attested by half a dozen or more editions of various extracts of Johnson's version of Paré's writings. Several of these productions include short synopses of Paré's life; since Packard (1926), however, no new attempt has been made to bring the whole story together again. Today, Paget's and Packard's *Lives* are out of print or difficult to obtain. Since there seems little hope that these books will be reprinted, it appears worthwhile to provide a new version of the story. I confess frankly that this book is the result of my protracted case of hero-worship; more important, it seems unfair that medical students and "young surgical apprentices" of our day should be denied an easily available source through which they too can be inoculated with my infection.

This book contains no truly new Paré material. I have translated all of Paré's *Case Reports and Autopsy Records* (Thomas, 1960) from Malgaigne and, where pertinent, have included examples of these here. All Paré *Lives* heretofore have mentioned some of the historical details of Paré's time, since these conditioned his life. To better understand Paré as a creature of his culture, it seemed worthwhile to present a little more of the political and basic medical material concurrent with the Paré story.

For the rapid orientation of the reader, a chronologic table has been prepared of the major events in France during Paré's lifetime, and a few events of general interest in the world of that period. A genealogic table is included, giving as much of the Paré family data as is available, and another of the Kings under whom he served.

Having made several trips to France to visit the scenes of Paré's experiences, I have been tempted to include a number of illustrations from that beautiful country. In reviewing other such attempts, however, these seem of dubious merit. Appearances are so ephemeral, especially in this rapidly changing age so remote from the period in point, that their presentation is hardly worthwhile. Pictures have been restricted to reproduction of an engraving of himself that Paré used in his first book on anatomy, and several maps.

Acknowledgments

I AM INDEBTED to many people helpful in the preparation of this book. The late Mrs. Hildegarde Shinners of Buffalo was tireless over years in several revisions of the manuscript, helping to make it more readable. My former secretary and friend, Mrs. Constance Crockett, of New York's East Aurora, has uncomplainingly retyped the manuscript several times.

In addition to the kind librarians of the Buffalo General Hospital, the University of Buffalo Medical School Library and of the Lockwood Memorial Library of the University of Buffalo, I have had much help from Miss Janet Doe and her successors at the Library of the New York Academy of Medicine, from the Grosvenor Library of Buffalo, the New York and the Cleveland Public Libraries, and from the Bibliothèque Nationale and the Musée Carnivalet of Paris. Dr. C. E. Kellett, of Newcastle, England, clarified several points concerning the *Anatomies* of Estienne and of de la Rivière. Mrs. Mildred Hoerr Lysle and her staff of the Editorial Department of the Cleveland Clinic Educational Institute have been most helpful in preparation of the manuscript for the press. Mr. Thomas Lanning and his staff of the Photographic Department of the Cleveland Clinic prepared the illustrations for the engravers.

W. B. H.

Chronology of Ambroise Paré and His Period

1510		Ambroise Paré born at Bourg-Hersent, Laval France.
1513		Ponce de Leon claimed Florida for Spain.
1515		François I crowned King of France; Henry VIII, King of England.
1520		Charles V elected Emperor, Holy Roman Empire. Capture of Mexico by Cortez.
1523		Paré apprenticed to Vialot, Master Barber-Surgeon of Vitré (tradition).
1527		Sack of Rome by Charles V.
1531		Paré apprenticed to barber-surgeon in Paris (tradition).
1533	(Approx.)	Paré started internship, Hôtel-Dieu.
		Vesalius to Paris to study anatomy with Sylvius.
1534		Jacques Cartier claimed Canada for France.
1535		Paré finished service at Hôtel-Dieu; started practice.
1536		Vesalius left Paris.
1537		Paré entered army service under Duke de Montejan; expedition to Turin. Discovered new treatment for gunshot wounds.
1538		Death of Montejan; Paré returned to Paris.
1541		Paré licensed as Master Barber-Surgeon.
	30 June	Married to Jeanne Mazelin.
1542		War between François I and the Emperor.
	Aug.	Paré to Perpignan with Vicount de Rohan.
	Sept.	Siege lifted, Paré to Paris.
1543		Publication of Vesalius' *Fabrica*.
		Birth of François, later King François II, to Henri and Catherine de' Médicis.
	June	Paré to Maroilles with de Rohan; to Landerneau; return to Paris.
1544		Paré writing book on gunshot wounds.
	Sept.	Boulogne taken by Henry VIII.
	Oct.	Paré to Landrecies under de Rohan, with François I.
1545	4 July	François, Paré's first child, baptized; short survival.
	Aug.	Publication Paré's *La Méthode de traicter les playes faictes par hacquebutes,* etc.
	Aug.	To Boulogne with de Rohan; wound of François de Guise.
1546		Étienne Dolet, publisher, burned for heresy.
1547	Feb.	Death of Henry VIII of England.
	31 Mar.	Death of François I.

	26 July	Coronation of Henri II at Reims.
		Dutch edition of Paré's *Gunshot Wounds*.
1548		Death of Jean Paré, barber-surgeon, of Vitré.
	June	Publication of Paré's *Anatomy, Briefve Collection*, etc.
	Aug.	Nephew Bertrand Paré, Jean's son, to live with Ambroise; unsuccessful attempt to educate him.
1550	Mar.	Boulogne ceded to France by England; Paré to Boulogne; Publication 2nd ed. of *Briefve Collection*.
	Sept.	Acquisition of Maison de la Vache and Meudon property.
1551		Negotiations of Henri II with German Protestant enemies of Charles V; background of Wars of Religion.
1552	March	2nd ed. of *Gunshot Wounds*, dedicated to Henri II.
	April	Paré with de Rohan to Toul, Nancy, Metz and Verdun.
	July	Capture of Damvilliers by Henry II; Paré's first use of ligature in amputations.
	26 July	Paré return to Paris.
	Aug.	Paré to Château-le-Comte with King of Navarre; return to Paris via Tournahan.
	30 Aug.	Paré to Reims, appointment as King's Surgeon-in-Ordinary.
	19 Oct.	Assault on Metz by Imperial troops.
	14 Nov.	de Rohan killed at St. Nicholas, near Nancy.
	8 Dec.	Paré smuggled into Metz with supplies.
	26 Dec.	Emperor abandoned siege of Metz.
1553	30 Jan.	Paré return to Paris.
	May	Emperor besieged Therouënne, near Boulogne.
	30 June	Fall of Therouënnne, Paré to Hesdin with defense. Siege of Hesdin, Paré in attendance.
	6 July	Death of Edward VI of England; Mary Tudor, Queen; married Philip of Spain.
	17 July	Fall of Hesdin; capture of Paré.
		Treatment of M. de Vaudeville; release; return to Paris.
1554	18 Aug.	Paré request for examination by College of Surgeons.
	23 Aug.	Preliminary examination passed.
	27 Aug.	Passed examination as Bachelor of Surgery.
	8 Oct.	Conference of Licentiate of College of Surgeons on Paré.
	3 Dec.	Licensed as "Sworn-Surgeon."
	17 Dec.	Admission to College of Surgeons as Master Surgeon; ridicule by Faculté de Médecine.
1555	31 Jan.	Death of Sylvius, aged 77.
	Oct.	Abdication by Charles V, sovereignty of Spain and the Netherlands to son Philip II.
1556	Jan.	Abdication as Emperor by Charles V to Ferdinand of Austria. Five year peace signed with France.
		War, France vs Spain in Italy.
1557	31 Jan.	War on France by Spain and England signed by Philip and Mary.
	10 Aug.	Battle of St. Quentin; French defeat by Duke de Savoy; capture of French leaders; Paré to La Fère to treat wounded.

CHRONOLOGY OF AMBROISE PARÉ AND HIS PERIOD

	20 Oct.	Duke de Guise made Lieutenant-General of France.
1558	1 Jan.	Attack on Calais by de Guise.
	6 Jan.	Fall of Calais.
	24 Apr.	Dauphin François married to Mary Stuart, niece of de Guise. Paré to camp at Dourlan; return to Paris.
	16 Nov.	Death of Mary Tudor; Elizabeth Queen of England, refused marriage to Philip II.
1559	3 Apr.	Peace signed between France and England.
	June	Marriage of Henri's daughter Elizabeth to Philip II, and his sister Marguerite to Duke de Savoy.
	29 June	Tournament injury of Henri II by Duke de Montgomery; treated by Paré and Vesalius.
	10 July	Death of Henri II; autopsy and embalmment by Paré. François II King of France.
	11 Aug.	Birth of Isaac, Paré's second child.
1560		Publication of French ed. of Vesalius' *Fabrica*.
	10 Mar.	Conspiracy of Amboise (Huguenots vs King) thwarted by de Guise.
	2 Aug.	Burial of Isaac Paré.
	30 Sept.	Baptism of Catherine Paré, third child.
	5 Dec.	François II died at Orleans; autopsy and embalmment by Paré; Mary of Scotland widowed. Charles IX King; Catherine de' Médicis Regent. Paré retained by King as Surgeon-in-Ordinary.
1561		Paré's move into Maison des Trois Maures.
	Apr.	Publication of Paré's *Anatomie universelle du corps humain*, dedicated to King of Navarre.
	15 Apr.	Charles IX crowned at Reims.
	4 May	Compound fracture of Paré's left ankle.
	Aug.	Return to Scotland of Mary, Queen of Scots, widow of François II.
	Sept.	Paré walking without a limp; much Catholic-Huguenot discord.
1562	28 Feb.	Publication of Paré's *La Methode curative des playes, & fractures de la teste humain*, etc.
	1 Mar.	Onset First War of Religion by "massacre" of Huguenots at Vassy and Sens. Philip sent aid to Catholics, Elizabeth sent aid to Huguenots under Conde and Coligny.
	Easter	Paré appointed Premier-Surgeon and Valet-de-Chambre by Charles IX.
	May	Paré to Bourges with the King. Plague and smallpox epidemic in Paris; 25,000 perished.
	Sept.	Siege of Rouen by Catholics.
	26 Oct.	Fall of Rouen; King of Navarre treated by Paré; died. Escape of Condé. Paré poisoned and recovered, on return trip to Paris.
	19 Dec.	Battle of Dreux won by Catholics; Paré treated wounded.
1563	18 Feb.	Assassination of Duke de Guise at Orléans; son Henri became third Duke de Guise.

	19 Mar.	Peace of Amboise, ending First War of Religion.
	July	Paré to Le Havre with combined French army against English.
	28 July	Fall of Le Havre to French.
1564	24 Jan.	Paré to Fontainebleau with the Court, to start two year tour of France with the King.
	3 Feb.	Publication of Paré's *Dix Livres de la chirurgie*, etc. First account of use of ligatures in amputations.
	13 Mar.	Start of Court tour from Fontainebleau, via Bar-le-Duc and Dijon to Lyon (13 June; Paré studied the plague.
	17 July	Arrival at Roussillon château; edict setting New Year's Day on 1 January.
	Autumn	Travel through Provence.
	Dec.	Christmas at Montpellier; Paré bitten by snake. French Huguenots began colonizing Florida.
1565	12 Jan.	Arrival of Court in Carcassonne.
	1 Apr.	Arrival in Bordeaux.
	29 May	Arrival at Bayonne. Conference French with Spaniards. Visit of Paré to Biarritz, observing whaling.
	12 July	Departure from Bayonne.
	14 Sept.	Arrival at La Rochelle; Huguenots rebellious.
	Nov.	Visiting Loire country.
	22 Dec.	Arrival at Moulins; Grand Assembly of Notables.
1566	Jan.	King Charles' attack of smallpox; median nerve injury during phlebotomy by Portail.
	Mar.	Visit to Clermont; experiment with bezoar.
	1 May	Return of Court to Paris.
1567		Paré's attempt to unite all surgery under one head; blocked by Faculté and College of Surgeons.
	Sept.	Outbreak of Second War of Religion.
	10 Nov.	Battle of St. Denis, won by Catholics; Constable paralyzed, treated by Paré to no avail.
1568		Publication Paré's book, *Traicte de la peste*, etc.
	13 Mar.	Battle of Jarnac; death of Condé.
1569	3 Oct.	Battle of Moncontour; Paré treating wounded at Plessis-les-Tours; expedition to Flanders; visit to Belgian cities.
	4 Nov.	Death Dr. Castellan, plague, at St. Jean-d'Angely.
	5 Dec.	Death Dr. Chapelain, same house, of plague. Paré to Paris.
1570		Paré divided his time between the Court and practice.
1572	Mar.	Publication Paré's *Cinq livres de chirurgie*.
	22 Aug.	Coligny shot in Paris, treated by Paré.
	24 Aug.	St. Bartholomew's Day Massacre of Huguenots in Paris; Paré protected in Louvre by the King.
1573		Publication Paré's *Deux livres de chirurgie*.
	4 Nov.	Death of Jeanne Mazelin Paré, aged 53, leaving Paré in charge of two teen-aged girls.
1574	18 Jan.	Marriage, Paré and Jacqueline Rousselet.
	30 May	Death Charles IX, aged 23, tuberculosis; autopsy and embalmment by Paré. Succession of Henri III.

CHRONOLOGY OF AMBROISE PARÉ AND HIS PERIOD xvii

		Paré appointed Premier-Surgeon, Councillor and Valet-de-Chambre.
1575	Jan.	Paré to Nancy to treat Duchesse de Lorraine; visit with fracture surgeon, Nicolas Picart.
	13 Feb.	Coronation of Henri III.
	Apr.	Publication Paré's *Les Oeuvres de M. Ambroise Paré*, dedicated to the King.
		Attempt by Faculté to ban publication; rejection of suit by Parlement.
	16 Apr.	Baptism of Anne, Paré's fourth child, first by Jacqueline Rousselet; lived until 1616.
1576	30 May	Son Ambroise baptized; Paré's fifth child, second by Jacqueline.
1577	1 Jan.	Foundation of Catholic League, headed by Henri, Duke de Guise.
	14 Jan.	Burial of infant Ambroise Paré.
	27 Mar.	Marriage of Jeanne Paré, Ambroise's niece and ward, to Claude Viart.
1578	6 Feb.	Marie Paré baptized; sixth child, third by Jacqueline.
	21 Mar.	Baptism of Claude Viart's son Ambroise; Paré godfather, support of Paré's questioned Catholicism.
	5 Apr.	2nd ed. manuscript of *Les Oeuvres* submitted to Faculté.
1579	8 Feb.	Publication Paré's *Les Oeuvres*, 2nd ed.
	8 Oct.	Baptism of Jacqueline Paré; seventh child, fourth by Jacqueline Rousselet.
		Drake claimed California for England.
1580	Mar.	New Religious Wars.
		Plague and influenza in Paris, killing 60,000 in six months.
		Paré on Plague Commission; reissue of 1568 *Book on the Plague*.
		Publication by Dean Gourmelen attacking Paré's surgical discoveries and practices. Paré began writing reply in his *Apologie and Treatise*, etc.
	31 Aug.	Injury of M. des Ursins, treatment by Paré, leading to writing of *Book on Mummy*, etc.
	3 Nov.	Drake completed circumnavigation of the globe.
1581	12 Feb.	Baptism of Catherine Paré; eighth child; fifth by Jacqueline.
	28 Mar.	Marriage of Catherine Paré, Jeanne Mazelin's third child, to François Rousselet, Jacqueline's brother.
1582	Jan.	Publication by Jacques Guillemeau of the third, Latin ed. of Paré's *Oeuvres*, as *l'Opera*.
	Mar.	Publication of *Discours d'Ambroise Paré*, etc., *De la Mumie*, etc. Contains best copper plate engraving of Paré at 72.
1583		Death of Claude Viart, husband of Jeanne Paré.
	8 Nov.	Baptism of Ambroise Paré III, ninth and last child, sixth by Jacqueline.
	10 Dec.	Paré still in practice; supervised amputation by assistant Daniel Poullet.
1584	June	Death of Duke d'Anjou, leaving Henri III last male of the Valois line.

	19 Aug.	Death of Ambroise III, the last of Paré's sons.
1585	13 Apr.	Publication 4th ed. of *Les Oeuvres*, the last seen through the press by Ambroise, containing the *Apologie and Treatise*.
	July	Eighth War of Religion, the "War of the Three Henris," Henri III, Henri de Navarre, and Henri de Guise.
1586		Mary Stuart imprisoned in London Tower.
1587		Man and woman burned for witchcraft in Paris.
	1 Mar.	News of execution of Mary Stuart; public mourning in Paris. Continuation of Religious Wars.
	1 July	Recording of Paré's will.
1588	11 Jan.	Marriage Jeanne Paré Viart to François Fôrest.
	Feb.	Temporary peace between Henri III and de Guise.
	9 May	Resumption of open warfare between King and Guise.
	11 July	Peace between King and Guise; Guise made Lieutennat-General.
	Aug.	Destruction of Spanish Armada by Drake. Catherine de' Médicis moved to Blois.
	12 Oct.	Henri III to Blois; Guise in control of France.
	16 Oct.	Meeting of States-General at Blois.
	23 Dec.	Murder of Guise at Blois by the King.
	24 Dec.	Murder of Cardinal de Guise at Bloise by the King.
1589	5 Jan.	Death of Catherine de' Médicis, aged 70, at Blois. Henri de Navarre fighting as Chief of Huguenot armies. Paré preparing 5th ed. of *Les Oeuvres,* published in 1598.
	1 Aug.	Assassination of Henri III by Jacques Clement; attended by Portail and Pigray; Paré absent because of age.
	1 Nov.	March on Paris by Navarre; defense by Catholic League.
1590	May	Siege of Paris by Navarre; misery in the city.
	July	Paré's meeting with Archbishop de Lyon; plea for peace.
	29 Aug.	Siege of Paris lifted.
	20 Dec.	Eve of St. Thomas; death of Ambroise Paré in his house.
	22 Dec.	Burial of Paré in St. André-des-Arts church.

Contents

	Page
Introduction	vii
Acknowledgments	xi
Chronology of Ambroise Paré and His Period	xiii
Prologue	3

Chapter
- I. Paré's Early Years and Environment (1510-1537) 10
  - The 16th Century Parisian Medical Scene 16
- II. Paré's Military Initiation (1537-1538) 26
  - Expedition to Turin (1537-1538) 28
- III. The Young Barber-Surgeon in Paris (1538-1542) 39
- IV. The Development of the Military Surgeon (1542-1552) 50
  - Boulogne 50
  - Boulogne 55
  - Damvilliers 62
  - Chateau-le-Comte 62
- V. King's Surgeon; The Great Sieges (1552-1553) 66
  - Metz 66
  - Hesdin 77
    - Two New Kings (1554-1562) 87
  - La Fère 90
  - Doullens (Dourlan) 92
    - 1560 96
    - 1561 97
    - 1562 101
- VII. Ambroise Paré, King's Premier-Surgeon (1562-1564) 103
  - Bourges 104
  - Rouen 104
  - Dreux 108
  - Le Havre 110

Chapter		Page
VIII.	Court Tour of France with Charles IX (1564-1566)	111
	1564	111
IX.	Civil War—Trip to Flanders—Surgical Writing (1566-1575)	131
	1567	131
	St. Denis	131
	1568	132
VI.	Court Surgeon in a Period of Civil Strife: Moncontour	134
	1570	140
	1572	141
	The St. Bartholomew's Massacre	142
	1574	146
	1576	149
X.	Les Oeuvres d'Ambroise Paré: The Final Years (1575-1590)	153
	Les Oeuvres d'Ambroise Paré	156
	1567	162
	1577	163
	1578	164
	1579	166
	Les Oeuvres, Second Edition	168
	1580	169
	1581	172
	1582	175
	1583	182
	1584	183
	1585	184
	1586	188
	1587	188
	1588	190
	1589	191
	1590	193
XI.	L'Apostille, A Post-script	195

Chapter	Page
The Paré Family	195
The Paré Property	198
Paré's Surgical Influence	203
The Paré Books: Chronology of his books appearing during his lifetime	207
Foot Notes	210
References	230
Index	233

AMBROISE PARÉ
Surgeon of the Renaissance

Prologue

A WAVE OF sound crackled through the forest, dry, intermittent, like a great fire in the distance. As the sound of fire in the woods silences bird song, so this one suddenly obliterated the dull background of a noise that had been so continuous as to have become ignored, the noise of an army on the march. In the sudden silence, the crackling grew in intensity and swelled in volume to a booming roar punctuated irregularly by the heavy percussion of small cannon. Now, a human element entered: the faint roars of men in fury, the exultant shouts of men triumphant, and the shrill screams of men suddenly clutched by unendurable agony.

The soldiers in the lead could see in the distance the scurrying approach of couriers returning from the advance guard which, with the scouts, had been leading King François' French army into Italy. For months, from the chill spring of 1537 into the warmth of summer, this army had marched eastward from Paris to Chambéry, and thence into the Alps. After crossing the river Ain below Bourges, it had labored through the foothills and toiled up the ever steeper slopes of Mount Cenis. The infantry had slogged its way under the load of steel helmets and breast plates, its burdens of pikes, battle axes and heavy arquebuses growing by the hour. Sweating horses and straining men had bulled the shambling supply carts and the more compact dead weight of the artillery pieces up long grades, and then hazardously braked them down the declines, as they slowly approached the Pass of Suza. There, they knew, the greatest toil would be over; the road then would be mainly downhill, down into warm and balmy Italy.

First the peal of slowly approaching bugles, and then the labored shouts of panting couriers brought them the news which the soldiers had already surmised. The Pass was occupied by the troops of Charles V, Emperor of the Holy Roman Empire. The French would have to fight their way through.

This was infantry business. Close combat with an entrenched foe armed with the newly perfected firearms was no fight for the mounted knights, who were leisurely approaching the Pass in all their gorgeous pageantry.

René, Duke de Montejan, as Colonel-General of Infantry, commanded the French foot soldiers. He sat his huge warhorse in the midst of his staff. Appraising the situation from the couriers' reports, he gave his orders to his subordinates, who dashed off to lead their detachments into the deadly business of the moment.

After the passage of the first few companies had somewhat eased the road congestion, Montejan sent for his surgeon. He smiled faintly as he watched the young man ride toward him. He had chosen Ambroise Paré from among several barber-surgeons who had applied for the job. Though this was the boy's first campaign, he was developing the attributes of a good army surgeon. Natural, of course, thought the Duke, for the young surgeon also was a Breton, and Bretons made good soldiers. Paré, in fact, came from Laval, a town in the Duke's own Anjou country. More important to the Duke, Paré had been trained well at the Hôtel-Dieu, that great charity hospital in Paris. Well-trained surgeons were hard to find; the Duke could teach him to be useful in war.

Ambroise rode up briskly. For one who had spent the last half of his 27 years confined to towns and hospitals, he rode well. The first few days on the road had been rather hard on him, but he had adjusted quickly to life in the saddle. He was sturdy and respectful, and he knew his own business. After saluting his chief, Paré dismounted and awaited his orders. The Duke smiled again as he looked down upon him; he was becoming quite fond of the young fellow.

"There will soon be a number of wounded who will need your help," the Duke said. "You will remain near me, but as soon as the first action is over, you may set up your equipment and help those who need you. Remount. We will go forward now."

Ambroise bowed and swung eagerly into the saddle. He wheeled his horse about and trotted back to rejoin the Duke's retinue. He and his assistant quickly checked over the surgical gear loaded on their pack mule. Then they cantered up briskly to join the Duke's guard, already on its way to the Pass.

The noise of the fight mounted, then gradually subsided. The cheers of victory were French and the French leaders rode forward eagerly to appraise the situation. But victorious cheers were not the only human sounds Ambroise heard. His ears were more attuned to the screams of the wounded. They lay in all postures of spent endurance; or, frantic in their fear and pain, floundered into the ditches to escape the flying hooves of the advancing horses. The great warhorses nimbly avoided the prostrate bodies upon which they might slip, but they lashed out in passing with deadly hooves at any man afoot before them. Paré and his assistant were at the trenches now. Bodies lay thicker there, and Montejan wheeled his horse to point out several gentlemen and officers who had fallen among their men. Paré and his assistant dismounted and quickly assessed their conditions. A few of the noble dead were of interest to the Colonel; their bodies were sent to the rear in carts. The lightly wounded were helped to mount and continued forward. A few severely wounded were put into carts to be brought forward to a spot where Ambroise could set up a rough aid station. Paré looked around him and saw that the common soldiers were being cared for by their fellows and by the women who had followed the infantry. The dead were stripped of their usable gear and left for burial. The battered and bruised were repaired roughly and helped on their way, to the rear or forward again.

The dislodged defenders of the Pass had retired to a little walled castle on a hillock in the midst of a wide meadow. The French swarmed out of the forest on the mountain slopes surrounding it and paused while their leaders decided strategy. Ambroise dismounted again, and he and his helper quickly set about treating the wounded brought up to them. Surgeons in the retinues of other noblemen joined them and soon the little clearing had been converted into a small outdoor operating room.

The bands of soldiers moved off on their assignments. A

challenge was sent to the castle by a group of mounted couriers. The defenders were offered freedom on surrender, death if assault were required. Their answer was an insult! The French would have to take the castle!

Observing a little elevation that overlooked the castle, one of the Captains, Le Rat by name, took a detachment to its summit. They set up a couple of culverins—long cannon with serpent-shaped handles—and soon were dropping balls of stone and iron that crashed into the castle and its outbuildings. The infantry advanced and the archers showered the foe's refuge with arrows. Under the protection of great mounted wooden shields, a battering ram lumbered up to the gates in the wall. Soon its measured, rhythmic clang swelled out even over the crackle of the guns, and within a few minutes the gate came crashing down. With exultant shouts, the infantrymen poured through the gap. Pike, sword, and battleaxe now rang on helmet and breastplate. The odds were too great for the outnumbered defenders. They withdrew into the keep of the castle, leaving the surrounding space filled with the enemy.

Montejan sent word back to Ambroise that he should come up and find shelter to set up his dressing station. Just then a group of horsemen arrived. Ambroise looked up to see them help Captain Le Rat dismount. The Captain limped painfully to a bench where he sat down and his friends lifted his left leg to extend it before him. Although pale, and obviously in much pain, his old gaiety had not quite left him. As the men slit and removed his fine leather boot, he quipped, "Well, after so long, today they got the Rat!"

Ambroise examined the injured leg. Wiping away the blood, he found that the wound wasn't as bad as it might have been. The ball, fired by some sharp-eyed harquebusier, had struck above the ankle, but had passed between the two leg bones without striking either of them. The Captain's leg could be saved.

Until today, Ambroise had had little experience with gunshot wounds. Most of the wounds he had seen in Paris had been inflicted with sharp or blunt instruments. None were really comparable with gunshot wounds. Arrow wounds approached nearest, but gunshot wounds were said to be poisoned. Even

Paré's respected medical authority, Jean de Vigo, had said so. De Vigo had detailed the proper treatment—cauterization of the wound with a red-hot iron or with boiling oil. Ambroise had learned the hot oil technic from other barber-surgeons, so he was ready to use it now.

The oil was bubbling in a little cauldron on the edge of Paré's brazier, where variously sized and shaped cauterizing irons nestled in their bed of glowing charcoal. Paré picked a few fragments of cloth and leather out of the wound where the ball had entered. He gradually worked his forceps into the wound, and finally its tip came out the other side. This made it easier; he wouldn't have to open a tract through the swollen flesh. He left his forceps in the wound, and with another picked up the end of a strip of linen soaking in the oil pot. He lifted it and snipped off a likely length. Dipping it once more to keep as much heat in it as possible, he lifted it over the wounded leg and let its end drop until he could grasp it in the jaws of the forceps extending through the ankle. Cautioning the Captain and the two men who were holding the leg, he quickly pulled the length of hot linen through the wound, leaving an end protruding from each side.

The Captain gasped and stiffened, swallowed hard, and then began breathing smoothly again. He managed a grin at Ambroise and complimented him on his dexterity. He had suffered wounds more painful than this, but never before one that had threatened to leave him walking on a peg-leg. After Ambroise had finished dressing the leg, he told the Captain how to take care of himself, promising to see him in the morning. Captain Le Rat was helped to his quarters by his attendants. In his later report of this case, Ambroise first made his famous comment on the successful outcome of a case, "Je le pensay, et Dieu le guarist"—I dressed him, and God healed him (Hamby, p. 161).

Paré and his assistant then hurriedly gathered up and packed their equipment and went looking for a sheltered spot to set up a more protected dressing station. The Imperial troops, realizing their hopeless situation, had called for a parley, and negotiations for a surrender were under way. Taking advantage of the interval, Ambroise sought shelter. He didn't want to go inside the castle's outer walls. Fighting might break out again, trapping him and his patients in a line of fire.

A hundred yards or so to the right of the castle gate was a moderate sized house that had been badly smashed in the conflict. Behind it was a barn with stone walls and a beamed and thatched roof that appeared to be fairly intact. Telling his assistant to await his signal, Ambroise walked over to inspect the house. He went around the corner of the barn and saw a covered shed attached to its side. Huddled in the straw there he found four dead soldiers. Propped against the rear wall were three more who were alive, but frightfully mangled and disfigured. They were unconscious, and their clothes still smoldered from powder burns.

Ambroise contemplated them narrowly. Obviously they had little longer to live; they were not suffering. Abruptly Ambroise sensed the presence of another. He turned to see a grey old soldier who had entered quietly and who also was evaluating the situation. The old man asked Paré if he thought the wounded men could be saved. Ambroise said that they soon would be dead. The old man stepped forward and bent over the first man. His shoulders swung slightly. Then he stepped astride the legs of the second. Meanwhile the first man had slipped flatter on the floor, gasped and gurgled and was still. The old soldier stepped over to the third man before Ambroise realized what had happened. The soldier then stood erect and wiped the blade of a short dirk he held in his right hand. He had cut the throats of the three wounded men. They were dead.

Ambroise cried out in horror. He berated the grizzled veteran for his cruelty. The soldier eyed him quietly, and calmly sheathed his dirk.

"Monsieur le chirurgien," he said, "you are young and perhaps have seen little of war. I have been in and out of it since I was a boy. There are worse things than dying; one can't die easier than this. I pray God that if I ever come to such a state, someone will be so kind as to do as much for me." So saying, he turned and walked out of the shed.

Ambroise shook his head, dazed by the impact of the things he had seen this day. The plight of the poor, dumb, helpless soldiers wrung his heart. He bitterly regretted ever having left Paris to witness such horrors. Yet, within him arose an overwhelming compassion. Perhaps he could do a little, in his own way, to ease the misery of unfortunates such as these. He tossed some straw over the seven still figures and stepped to the corner of the barn. With a whistle, he called his assistant.

Such was his introduction into the military medical service that was to become the pattern of life for Ambroise Paré, the man who became the Father of French Surgery. What had been its past? How would Paré influence its future?

CHAPTER I

Paré's Early Years and Environment
1510-1537

THE RENAISSANCE BLOOMED in France in the 16th century, almost a century later than in Italy, from which it came. Its influence spread throughout Europe gradually and fitfully, affecting different countries in different ways according to the resistance of the people in clinging to their old ways, and the resistance of their rulers to change. It touched the separate components of society variously, varying in times and places. In medicine and in surgery, response to the startling stimulus of the Renaissance came later than it did in art and architecture. As a matter of fact, in France the influence of the Renaissance did not reach its peak until the 19th century. On the rolls of the pioneers of the new spirit in surgery, the name of the 16th century Ambroise Paré shines with outstanding brilliance.

In the little village of Bourg-Hersent, outside the walled town of Laval, in the French provence of Mayenne, Ambroise Paré was born early in the 16th century, only a few years after Columbus discovered America. The precise date of his birth is unknown and will remain so until perhaps some lucky accident brings to light the documentary dating of it that has eluded many careful searchers for more than three and a half centuries. Paré himself was inconsistent in referring to his age.[1] It is quite likely that he did not know his exact birth date, or else did not consider it a matter of great importance. I have accepted the date of 1510, recorded at the time of his death by Pierre de l'Estoile, an on-the-scene reporter, although de l'Estoile could hardly have been expected to know more about it than Ambroise himself.

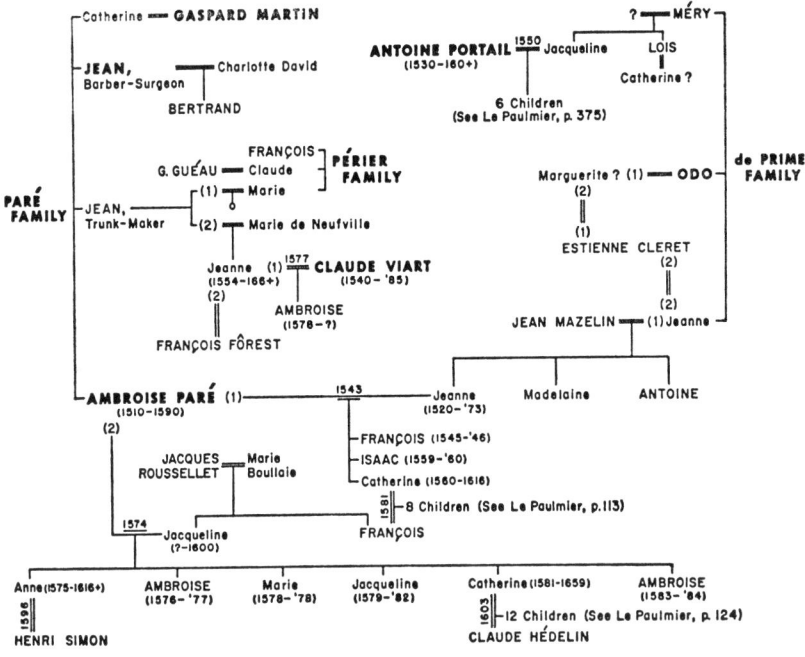

Figure 2. Genealogy of the Paré family.

Nothing certain is known of Ambroise's antecedents. We only have the information that he himself left us in his writings, and some information about his contemporaries and relatives gleaned from old legal documents by the historian Le Paulmier. Ambroise's father, whose first name is unknown, has been thought to have been either a cabinet-maker, or a barber-surgeon and valet to Guy XVI,[2] the Duke de Laval. Jean, one of Ambroise's brothers, was a trunk-maker who moved to Paris and had a shop in the rue de La Huchette. Another brother, also named Jean, was a master barber-surgeon who practiced in the Brittany town of Vitré. A sister, Catherine, married Gaspard Martin, a master barber-surgeon who practiced in Paris. It seems more likely that this close attachment for barber-surgery would have developed in the children of a barber-surgeon rather than in the off-spring of a cabinet-maker. Ambroise himself has left us no clue. He wrote of his barber-surgeon brother but not of his brother-in-law. He might not have had reason to mention the work of his father

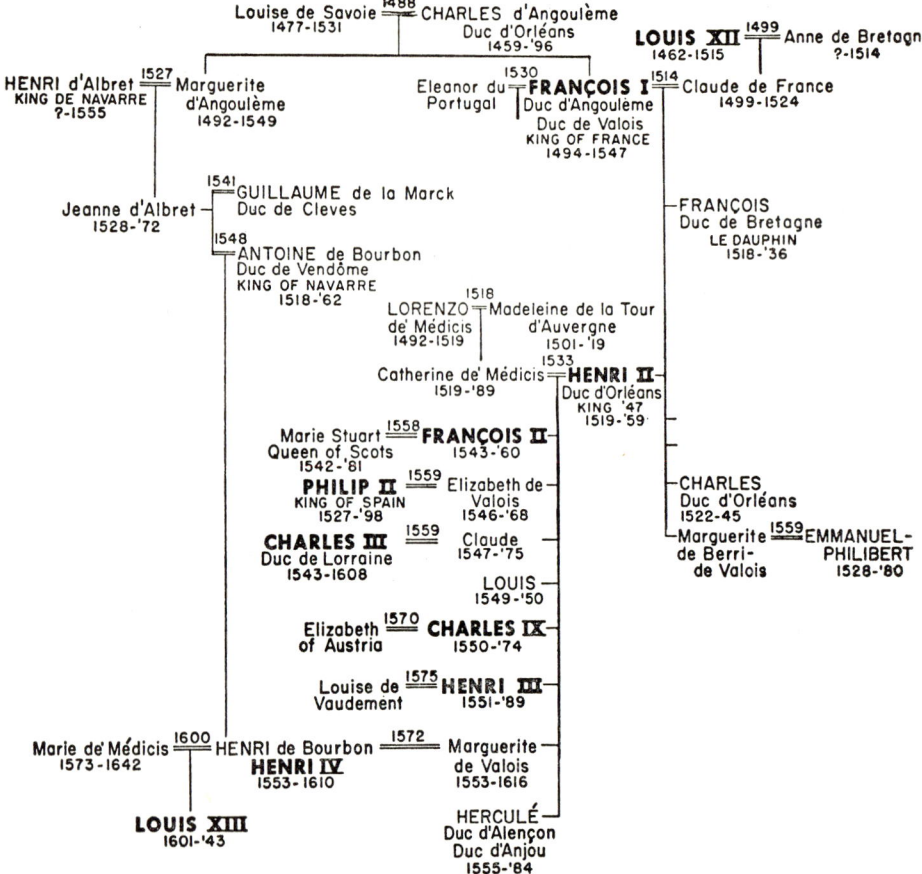

Figure 3. Valois-Bourbon genealogy.

in any event. These family data are taken chiefly from Le Paulmier. Malgaigne, Paré's greatest biographer, was unaware of them. Malgaigne also was confused by material furnished him by Dr. Émile Bégin of Metz, another of Paré's attempted biographers, of whom more will be said later.

Bourg-Hersent is now a part of the town of Laval. A two-storied, timber and stucco house at #82 rue du Ponceau bears a plaque proclaiming it to be the birthplace of Ambroise Paré. Turner, the French historian, said that this house is a 19th century reconstruction of the original that had practically fallen apart by the time it was re-built. It is roughly a half-mile from the old chateau-fortress on the right bank of the Mayenne River, where Guy XVI ruled the provence as Duke de Laval when Ambroise was a boy. The Duke had three wives; in 1517, the Duchesse was Anne de Montmorency (not to be confused with her brother, the Constable, who, peculiarly enough, had the same name). Their oldest son Claude, on the death of his father in 1531, became Duke Guy XVII, and took Ambroise riding through Brittany to a campaign in 1543. This duke married Claude de Foix, daughter of the Marshal d'Odet; we shall read of her later.

Little is known of Ambroise's youth. A number of legends and romances have developed about it, but in his methodical way Malgaigne has deflated most of them. Paré himself regretted in print on more than one occasion that he had not had more education, especially the opportunity of learning Greek and Latin, necessary preliminaries for the standard study of medicine and surgery at the time. However, perhaps if he had enjoyed a better education, he might have simply become another unknown doctor of his generation; his very handicaps assisted him. How, when, where, and under whom he served his apprenticeship in barber-surgery is unknown. It is probable that he had some of his training in the provinces before he went to Paris around 1530, at the age of 20. He has only told us (Malgaigne, III, p. 46; Hamby, p. 116) that in 1525, when he was in Angers with his brother Jean, he saw a beggar pretending to have a gangrenous arm which he used to stimulate the flow of alms from people visiting the church. While Paré watched, the arm fell from beneath the cloak where it had been fastened. In retrieving it, the beggar revealed two perfectly good arms; the gangrenous one had been stolen from a hanged corpse. He was condemned by the magistrate to be lashed, with the arm hanging from his neck, and was banished from the country. Ambroise then described two other instances of his brother Jean's unmasking of such mendicants. These reports give grounds for suspecting that Ambroise might have been his brother's barber-surgeon apprentice.

With some training already behind him, Paré went to Paris

about 1530 and presumably worked under another barber-surgeon there. The record contains no note of the circumstances. Another brother, Jean the trunk-maker, lived there with his wife Marie Périer, as did his sister Catherine with her husband, the barber-surgeon Gaspard Martin. Paré must have kept in touch with these close relatives, if indeed he did not live with one of them, for judging from the record, throughout his life he loved and lived closely with his friends and relations.

The walled city of Paris into which Paré now moved contained some 150,000 people. Historians estimate that six or seven thousand of them were paupers. The bubonic plague was raging, as it did periodically within the close confines of all the old walled cities; the mortality was high. Under the stimulus of the young king, François I,[3] the face of the city was changing. The Louvre was being converted from a medieval fortress into a Renaissance palace. The Hôtel-de-ville and St. Eustace's great church were under construction. Nôtre-Dame,[4] the Sainte-Châpelle, the Hôtel-Dieu,[5] and the Grand Châtelet,[6] the grim fortress-prison on the north bank of the Seine, were the major landmarks of the city. The Ile-de-la-Cité[7] was still the important center of town and only the bridges joining it to the mainland spanned the Seine at the time. The river's entrance to the city was guarded on the left bank by the Tournelles Castle. Downstream, the Tour de Nestle[8] guarded the left bank and the Louvre the right. Between the Tour du Coin (Corner Tower) of the Louvre and the Tour de Nestle stretched a great chain barrier supported on floating masts. It could be lowered at will to arrest river traffic. The Hôtel de Nestle, of which the Tower was a part, lay within the city walls built by Philippe-Auguste in 1200. This site in now occupied by the Institute and the Mint.

The part of the city on the left bank of the Seine was enclosed by the wall of Philippe-Auguste. This defense line stretched southeastward from the Tour de Nestle roughly along a route now traced by the rues Mazarin, des Écoles and Le Moine, ending eastwardly at the river at about the Pont-du-Sully. On the right bank, the city had outgrown the old walls but was enclosed within those built in 1358 by Étienne Marcel. This wall started at the river at about the present Boulevard Bourdon,

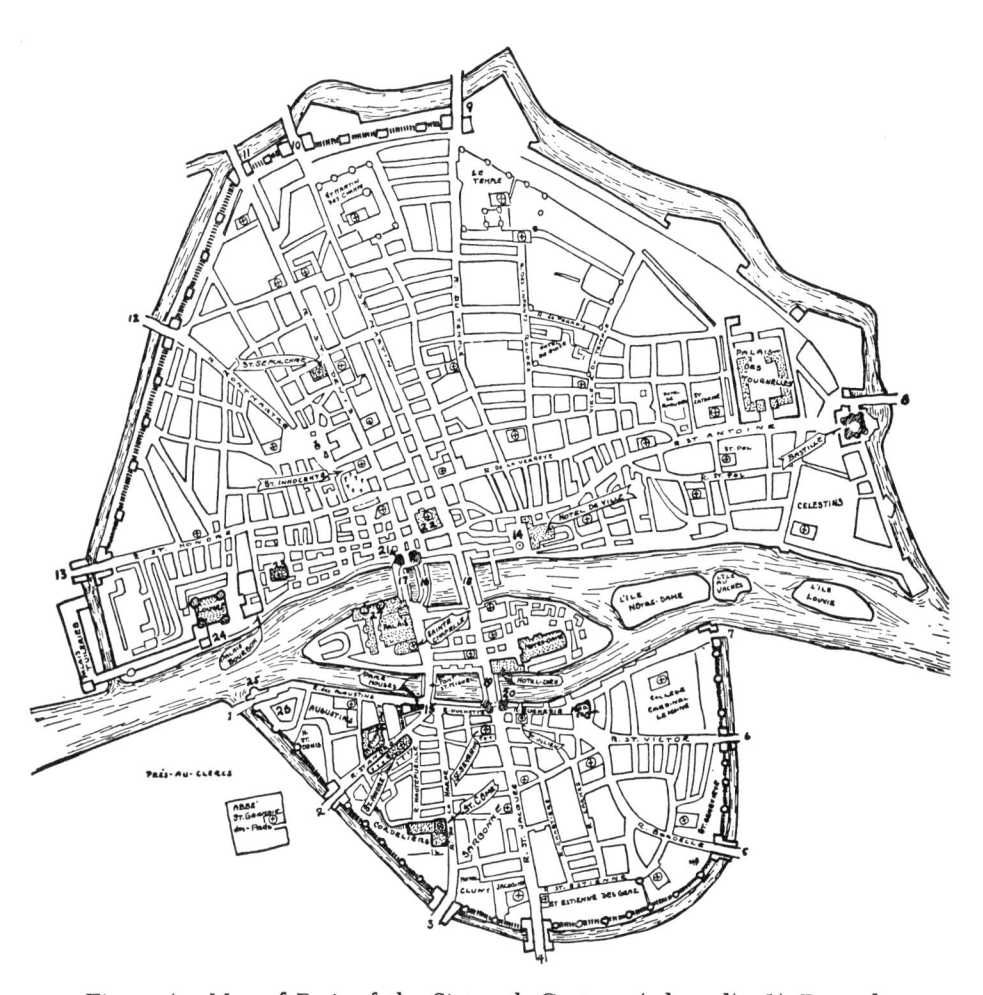

Figure 4. Map of Paris of the Sixteenth Century (adapted): 1) Porte de Nestle; 2) Porte de Bucy; 3) Porte St. Michel; 4) Porte St. Jacques; 5) Porte de Bordelle; 6) Porte St. Victor; 7) Porte de la Tournelle; 8) Porte St. Antoine; 9) Porte du Temple; 10) Porte St. Martin; 11) Porte St. Denis; 12) Porte de Montmartre; 13) Porte St. Honoré; 14) Place de Grève; 15) Place St. Michel; 16) Pont-au-Change; 17) Pont-aux-Marchants; 18) Pont Nôtre-Dame; 19) Petit Pont; 20) Petit-Châtelet; 21) Grand-Châtelet; 22) Church St. Jacques de la Boucherie; 23) Church St. Germain l'Auxerrois; 24) Tour du Coin; 25) Tour de Nestle; 26) Hôtel de Nestle; 27) la Conciergerie.

enclosed the Bastille, extended along the present Boulevards Beaumarchais, du Temple, St. Martin and St. Denis, then curved south-eastward along the rue d'Aboukir, then southerly to reach the Seine at about the Pont-du-Carrousel.

The streets of old Paris were narrow, only six to twenty feet in width. They were usually unpaved, although some of the major ones were cobble-stoned. Sewage disposal was elementary. Wastes usually were thrown from windows into shallow ditches along the curbs. In wet weather, the streets were filthy quagmires, and in hot weather the city literally stank. Paving was being extended as rapidly as possible, but the Parlement had many demands on its funds, and taxation was exorbitant. The nobility lived largely out of town; in inclement weather, they deserted the city completely. Their town houses were small estates called *hôtels,* enclosed within walls to keep out the populace, and almost as impregnable as fortresses. Travel was usually on foot or on horseback. No carriages were allowed in Paris until its streets had been gradually widened. Before the reign of Henri III,[9] only two carriages were permitted in the city—one for the Queen and one for the Queen-Mother, Catherine de'Médicis.[10] Chairs supported on poles toted by porters carried the frail, the infirm, and those averse to horseback.

THE 16TH CENTURY PARISIAN MEDICAL SCENE

Prior to the 10th century, the Western World really had no medical or surgical knowledge except folklore. Beginning with the School of Salerno in Italy in the 11th century, schools arose under Church protection and support. They were almost exclusively devoted to clerical and general educational disciplines. At Salerno, Arabic medical manuscripts first were translated into Latin. Because they were laboriously handcopied, diffusion of the information contained in them was very slow. The 13th century saw the development of universities in Italy. Some of their doctors, originally doctors of philosophy, began specializing in translating medical writings from the Arabic, and imparting their knowledge to others. These doctors were churchmen. Only gradually did they begin considering themselves to be doctors of medicine. The highest type of research thought possible—and the quickest way to fame—was to find and translate a previously unknown Arabic manuscript into Latin. Such texts being rare, the next best form of medical achievement for these monks was to compile treatises as complete as possible on all phases of medicine from fragmentary sources.

While these writers and teachers did use their knowledge for the benefit of the sick, such practice of medicine distinctly was held by them to be a diversion and an intrusion into their scholarly endeavors. Almost all of the universities made their candidates for medical degrees swear never to do any manual work, which automatically excluded them from the field of operative surgery.

In the 14th century, the Italian universities lost the support of the Church because the Popes had moved to Avignon in France, and the French universities then became pre-eminent. Montpellier was the most important, although that of Paris was growing rapidly. Medicine had not previously been a serious pursuit there. But, with greater affluence derived from closer proximity to the Holy See, the French schools could afford more manuscripts, and so study developed a healthy spurt of growth. Guy de Chauliac[11] became especially interested in surgery, stimulated by the "new" ideas found in the recently discovered writings of the ancient Greeks, Hippocrates[12] and Galen.[13]. Disregarding the university strictures, Guy practiced manual surgery, as indeed a few of his predecessors had done.

By the 15th century, rag paper making and printing from movable type were invented in the West, and learning no longer remained the exclusive possession of those universities wealthy enough to buy expensive manuscripts. Since the end of the 14th century, the most learned scholars had ceased translating the Arabic writers and had begun to study the Greek and Latin authors who antedated them. A rich store of these manuscripts was found collecting dust in convent and monastery libraries, and now printed copies and French and Latin translations were widely dispersed throughout western Europe.

Another tremendously important event made its impact indirectly upon medicine at that time. Heretofore, all recourse had been to authority, and the oldest authority was considered necessarily the best. Then Columbus discovered America, opening a whole new concept of thought, as well as of physical phenomena. There was no authority for this new entity and the early 16th century thinker perforce became his own authority. This attitude invaded medicine, and experience and rationality began challenging authority. But it was not a conceded point; those in authority still defended their positions bitterly against every attack and encroachment.

In the early 16th century, when Paré was born, France was still in a terminal state of transition from a collection of medieval baronial fiefs into an integrated country. French medicine and surgery were no more cohesive. The practitioners of each city guarded their prerogatives and owed allegiance to no central authority, although they all drifted into a similar pattern. The medical profession in Paris was under the nominal control of both the Crown and the Parlement.[13a] It was divided sharply into three classes. Controlling the medical schools were the physicians—the patricians of the lot—jealously guarding the rights and privileges of the Faculté de Médecine. Candidates for the study of medicine came from the universities; they were churchmen who had learned the classics, Latin, Greek, mathematics and church matters. Their medical instruction was in Latin; they studied the classical writings of Hippocrates, Galen, the Arabs and other accepted authorities. There was little contact with patients; the students' questions of why and how were answered from the books—if the books had the answers. Anatomy and surgery were taught theoretically. Practical experience was considered to be fraught with chance and error. Many students graduated without ever having seen a dissection; a very rare few ever participated in one. The texts available contained few if any illustrations; since even these were very crude, mental visualization of hidden parts depended entirely upon verbal exposition. Medical writing in the vernacular was frowned upon because this laid information open to uneducated eyes. Indeed, there was not even a true French language; each district spoke its own dialect, although a basic patois had developed. It was common for the traveled and the educated to be better able to understand people from neighboring foreign countries than those from adjoining French provinces. Later in the century

Ronsard,[14] Rabelais, Montaigne and other writers led in establishing the basic French language. While no educated person would want to write in the vulgar tongue, the Faculté had the legal authority to prevent the publication of medical writing of which it did not approve. Beyond the adverse effects of the restrictions imposed by the compulsory communication in Latin, the policy did have one great merit; the medical people of the civilized world had a common language. To moderns, this would seem a tremendous boon.

After graduation, the physician was an exalted person and was required to comport himself as such. He wore the "Long Robe" and viewed his patients distantly. He might not see them at all; instead, he might diagnose from observation of a sample of the patient's urine and from reported symptoms, comparing the list with the writings of the ancients. If he were mathematically inclined, he would be intrigued with the exciting field of astrology and might fit this superstition into his medical practice. Even Jean Fernel[15] devoted twelve years or more, and more money than he could afford, to this distraction before discarding it. The physician kept his hands clean and touched no medical instrument. If a boil needed opening, he called in a barber-surgeon who lanced it under the physician's supervision. If a graver problem presented itself to him, he called a more experienced surgeon who operated under his direction. He might botanize and even compound his own drugs if he chose, or if it interested him to do so, but usually an apothecary relieved him of this drudgery. To compensate for these privileges, the physician was bound under oath to do no manual work; to give a certain amount of his time to the poor; to serve his turn of duty during epidemics, although he could hire others to do this for him; and, if he kept up his university connections, to teach poor scholars at reduced rates. His privileged existence eventually led to indolence and sterility.

In the universities, surgery was only a branch of therapy, and the physician got lay assistance, usually from a barber, to do the simple operations he required, such as draining abscesses, opening boils, or drawing blood from a vein. Because the Arabs had done no operative surgery, operative surgery constituted no part of the art of medicine when it was transplanted to Western Europe. Surgery was a field despised both by the physicians and by the fastidious. Such scorn was not surprising in an age before asepsis, when infection took a forbidding toll; and before anesthesia when agony was almost invariably the swift result of all surgery and heavy restraint was required for any but the most trivial of operations. Only the extremely compassionate, or the extremely strong-willed, or the sadistic could stomach the necessary accompaniments. Surgery was the therapeutic resource solely of those sufferers under the direct threat of death or else in such deep misery that more could be tolerated only in strong hope of relief. It is a tribute to the boundless optimism of humanity that any man of good will and superior mental capacity would enter the field at that time. Even in those authoritarian days, however, not all patients with strangulated hernias, broken bones, and bladders obstructed with stones were content to die under purely verbal incantation, oral medication or spiritual ministration. Some desperate characters impelled skillful manual workers to cut them open and get at the lesion. Sufficient success attended these fumbling beginnings for some laymen to repeat doing the particular operations at which they had succeeded until they became adept at them. Requiring assistance, they took on apprentices who learned their masters' methods and eventually began operating independently. There were not enough patients with a specific ailment requiring operation in any one particular community to keep such a specialist busy, so they wandered from town to town operating wherever they could find patients. To find such patients they became advertisers and frequenters of fairs where people accumulated periodically. Human nature being what it is, the claim to perform life-saving operations also inevitably attracted the deceitful, who pretended skills they didn't have to cheat those in dire need. The charlatans unfortunately out-numbered the conscientious in this new field. So there developed outside the universities a group of primitive surgeons with whom educated physicians would have no dealings.

It is difficult to trace the development of true surgery in Paris. Malgaigne (Intro., p. cxx) exhaustively studied the evidence at hand without satisfying himself as to the exact sequence of development. From the earliest days of the healing arts, laymen had performed some manual surgery, independently, or at the behest of physicians. Being skilled with the razor, the barber was the logical person to perform minor operations; this was what happened in most primitive societies. Some barbers or other mechanics became bone-setters and handled the mechanical requirements in cases of fractures. Eventually these practioners banded together into guilds or trade unions to protect their prerogatives. The Corporation of Barber-Surgeons of Paris was mentioned officially as early as 1301 (Paget, p. 23). By the time Paré arrived upon the scene, it was a strong group. Its members were licensed to practice after serving an apprenticeship and taking two examinations. Their Chief was the King's Premier Barber-Surgeon, and they made their vows and paid their annual devotions in the Church of St. Sepulchre in rue St. Denis. Their patron saints were Sts. Cosmo and Damien, martyred medieval surgeons. Indeed, these saints were shared with the true surgeons as well. To earn the title of Master Barber-Surgeon, they passed examinations and paid a fee to the Faculté de Médecine. They were obligated to dissect in the Medical School for the physicians, and to renew their vows annually on St. Luke's Day.

Those who aspired to be licensed as barber-surgeons were not educated people. They served apprenticeships under barber-surgeons, and their lives were hard ones. They slaved in the barber-shops, shaving patrons, trimming beards, clipping hair, dressing wigs, and assisting their masters in their crude surgery. Their masters were not eager to have these potential competitors learn much or progress rapidly; they were kept at their menial tasks as rigorously as possible. Apprentices with ambition, intelligence and energy to learn and to progress in surgery had few literary resources. Unable to read Latin, they had to depend upon word-of-mouth instruction and whatever French translations of earlier authors were available to them. It is unlikely that many apprentices were able to afford them. Guy de Chauliac's was the first such book. Paré often referred to advice taken from "the good Guidon," as he called de Chauliac. Later, a French translation of Jean de Vigo[16] was published at Lyon by

Nicolas Godin in 1525 and was reprinted in Paris in 1530. In the 16th century, lectures for the apprentices were given by physician instructors at the Medical School, but they were given in Latin, which the apprentices unfortunately couldn't understand. In 1491 (Malgaigne, Intro., p. cxlviii), the surgeons complained to the Faculté that some of the instructors were teaching barbers' apprentices in French. Three years later the Faculté got around to replying; on 11 January 1494 they declared that the instructors henceforth would be ordered to read Guy de Chauliac and other authors in Latin; would "give certain explanations in the familiar French tongue as they judged proper"; and also would teach the apprentices anatomy. For this purpose, the apprentices were permitted to buy a body exposed on the gibbet. The lectures were probably perfunctory exercises by obligated, uninterested, and uninspired instructors, but the surgeons were jealous of any instruction given their competitors. To avoid taking apprentices away from their masters' shops during business hours, which ran from dawn into the night, the professors "out of the goodness of their hearts" gave the lectures to these tired lads at four o'clock in the morning (Malgaigne, Intro., p. ccxxx). Such was an apprenticeship in Paris; Paré was lucky if he had the chance to serve most of his in the provinces.

Between the university doctors and the barber-surgeons existed another class of surgeons. They may originally have been university-educated men who took up manual surgery prohibited by their university oaths, or simply more ambitious barber-surgeons who took courses at the university. In a royal ordinance of 1311, Phillipe-le-Bel regulated their activities, placing them under the jurisdiction of his Premier Barber-Surgeon, Jean Pitard. This royal regulation probably was the real origin of the Confraternity of Saint-Côme, whose members were sworn at the Châtelet to their duties. They were known as *Chirurgiens-juré*, sworn-surgeons, and were given the title of Master Surgeon. Before being admitted to the title, they were required to take a prescribed apprenticeship. It is interesting to note that as late as Paré's time, two centuries after, their list never held more than a dozen or so names.

Ever eager to close the cultural gap that separated them from the physicians, the surgeons of the Confraternity of St. Côme wheedled the Faculté for years to be admitted to the University. In the 16th century, they were delighted to be received as "scholars of the Faculté." Their delight was tinged with dismay, however, when they discovered that these terms were literal; the surgeons had to sit the benches in the Medical School, and to learn to read and to speak Latin. Candidates to the Confraternity thereafter had to come up through the University before being admitted. The surgeons of the Confraternity then aspired to recognition as a School of Surgery ranking with the Faculté de Médecine. Quite unofficially from the University's standpoint, they thereupon set up their own school, which they called the College of Surgery of St. Côme, in connection with the church of St. Côme. Their very building, reconstructed in 1707 after the original had collapsed, according to Le Grand, still stands on the south side of the rue de l'École de Médecine, near the Boulevard St. Michel. Presently, it houses the School of Languages of the University of Paris. The University never admitted the College of St. Côme to rank with the Faculté de Médecine, and eventually forced it to end its pretences of university quality. The major fault of the Sworn-surgeons was that, while aping the customs and jealous of the prerogatives of university rank, they were unwilling to give up their trade status and to submit to university authority and discipline. On the other hand, they were envious of the barber-surgeons and harrassed them at every opportunity, so that the Faculté often supported the barbers against them in court actions. They were especially irritated at being forced to practice under the ultimate control of the King's Premier Barber-Surgeon, which menial status was encouraged by the Faculté de Médecine to help keep the surgeons in their place.

Ambroise Paré came to Paris between 1530 and 1533, and probably worked again as an apprentice in a barber shop. The training available could not satisfy one of his temperament and soon—again the date is unknown—he entered the Hôtel-Dieu as a "compagnon-chirurgien," a status somewhat akin to that of the modern Intern. If 1533 was the date, it was the same year in which the 19-year-old Vesalius [17] came from Brussels to study anatomy with Sylvius. The Hôtel-Dieu was the only public hospital in Paris. Paré found plenty of work to do, to which he referred proudly throughout his life.

The Hôtel-Dieu was an ancient place, founded some time around 660 by St. Landry, the 28th Bishop of Paris (Chevalier). It was enlarged by St. Louis[18] about 1227 and was supported by his successors, but it was chronically overcrowded. It is interesting that the latest addition to the institution, the Hall of Legat, had been donated by Antoine Cardinal DuPrat, just before Paré began working there. This was a ward with a beautiful Renaissance facade facing westward at the end of the Petit-Pont. Even this addition did not end the congestion. During King François' imprisonment in Madrid after the loss of the battle of Pavia in 1525, the Cardinal was the King's Chancellor. He became so wealthy that he aspired to be Pope, and offered a huge bribe to facilitate his elevation. On the King's return home, he investigated the Cardinal, confiscated his wealth, and ruined him. Sharing his ruin was one of his clerks, Jean Mazelin, father of Jeanne, the girl who later became Ambroise's wife.

In this period, the Hôtel-Dieu was a collection of buildings of various ages standing on the south side of the island beside the Parvis, or Place Nôtre-Dame. Engravings of the time showed that it even partly overlapped the corner of the western facade of the Cathedral. After being damaged by fires on many occasions, the building finally burned down in the 19th century. The plot being inadequate and the site making the building obscure the view of the Cathedral, it was rebuilt in its present location across the island between 1868 and 1878. Its original site is marked now by the riverside grass plot bearing the statue of Charlemagne.

The old hospital was served originally by a group of Catholic lay-brothers and sisters sworn to the service of the poor, without attachment to any single Order. They chose the ablest one among them to be their head, giving him the title of Master of the Hôtel-Dieu. In 1505, according to Rousselet, the administration became so chaotic and the patient care so negligent that the Parlement named a "Commission of Eight" citizens to take over the temporal management of the hospital. The care of the sick was the duty of the Brothers and Sisters, and they undertook to carry care of patients even into their homes. Abuses of this "out-patient service" became so flagrant that in 1535 a new Parlement order deprived them of this privilege. As early as 1327, Charles-le-Bon[19] had ordered the two physicians of the Châtelet to visit the sick in the Hôtel-Dieu and gave them a number of medical students to assist them in their duties. The religious group opposed these reforms and certain of their numbers were removed from service. Some of the students who participated in the dispute were jailed.

Probably most of the students in attendance were young barber-surgeon apprentices; how Ambroise obtained his appointment is not known. He himself has told us that he studied sick people, assisted at operations, did some operations himself, did autopsies, and dissected for the professors. This was rather remarkable training for a surgeon of the time, for even the most superficial dissection had only recently been permitted. During this period, Paré decided to write an anatomy for barber-surgeons; he and a friend, Thierry de Héry, began preparing dissections as a groundwork for it. The two went through their examinations together and were together when licensed as Master Barber-Surgeons in 1541, according to Le Paulmier (p. 22). Singularly, in none of his voluminous writings did Paré mention any physician or surgeon under whom he worked, nor any of his other companions on the service. This is strange, since later he always listed to the last man all of those who saw patients with him. Perhaps this last detail was simply a way of indicating to his readers that his statements could be verified by asking those mentioned; routine case reports, earlier used by Hippocrates, were matters to be redeveloped centuries later.

CHAPTER II

Paré's Military Initiation
1537-1538

Paré finished his service at the Hôtel-Dieu in about 1536; again he was not consistent in his reports of his years of service. One must remember, however, that various years at that time were not uniform in length and might fluctuate between eight and sixteen months.[20] In the later years of so tumultuous a life, one might be forgiven for miscounting. Menegaux said that Paré was *compagnon-chirurgien* from 1530 to 1536, but this also was an estimate; no records exist from the time. At any rate, Paré did not then take the examinations that would have permitted, and that were required for, him to practice independently. Whether he worked as an assistant to an established practitioner, or whether something else caused the delay, we do not know. Our next record finds Paré on his way to Italy with the army in 1537. Thus, he set the pattern he would follow through his entire life: Parisian civil practice and following the wars. Paget has suggested that Paré might have been too poor to pay the fees for examination then. This hardly seems the only reason. The fees were not large, and even after returning from Italy wealthy enough to do other things more expensive, he delayed another three years before taking the examinations.

Ambroise Paré's fame developed chiefly from his discoveries made as a military surgeon. The political epoch into which he was born provided full scope for one talented in this role. The 16th century opened with three ambitious and able young men on the most important thrones in Europe. Henry VIII (1419-1547) became King of England in 1509, François I (1494-1547) King of France in 1515, and Charles V[21] (1500-1558) King of

Spain in 1516, of Austria and Burgundy in 1519, and Emperor of the Holy Roman Empire in the same year. As a result of conflicting and overlapping inheritances of property and disputed authority, as well as of unbridled greed for power, the three quarreled and fought together through their entire lifetimes and left heritages of dispute to generations of their successors.

In the spring of 1537, Ambroise was in practice of some sort in Paris, out of his hospital service, but not yet licensed. At this moment, the King sent an expedition against Turin, the modern Torino, in the Italian Piedmont. The army was under the command of the Grand-Master, Anne de Montmorency.[22] Henri the Dauphin went with him, learning the art of war. Next in rank was Claude d'Annebault.[23] René, Duke de Montejan[24] was Colonel-General of Infantry; he needed a barber-surgeon to accompany him. How Ambroise obtained the appointment we do not know. Anjou was the territory of which Angers was the ancient capital. Since Abroise had been there as a boy, and his brother practiced at nearby Vitré, the Duke might have heard of him through a friendly intercessor. At any rate, Paré was given the job and embarked on his first military experience.

In the 16th century, the army had no coordinated service departments. Each commander took the field responsible only for his personnel. Little attention was paid to the welfare of the common soldier. Charles-the-Bold, Duke of Burgundy in the time of Louis XI (1461-1483), had made some attempt to organize a medical service, attaching a surgeon to each company of 800 men, but the innovation had not been followed up. Now, each nobleman took along in his retinue a staff of servants, physicians, surgeons, and barber-surgeons adequate for his needs. Barbers, charlatans, and female camp-followers went along entirely unofficially, serving the troops for whatever they could command in the way of fees. Paré told us specifically that he went as a surgeon of the Duke, and not as an independent camp-follower. In certain instances, commanders would send their especially skillful surgeons to help their friends in time of need, or a nobleman would pay such a surgeon privately to care for some member of his retinue.

Expedition to Turin (1537-1538)

Turin, or Torino, is in the Piedmont section of Italy; the route from Paris runs via Lyon and over the Alps. Although Montejan commanded the Infantry, noblemen did not march. They and their retinues traveled in the saddle. It is probable, then, that on his first campaign, Ambroise, long a city dweller, had to become inured to life on horseback. From Fontainebleau to Lyon, the road traverses beautiful country, becoming increasingly hilly, with lovely vistas of rolling farm land. In those days, the hill tops were crowned with castles. Paré told the story of their progress in his *Apologie*, written retrospectively in

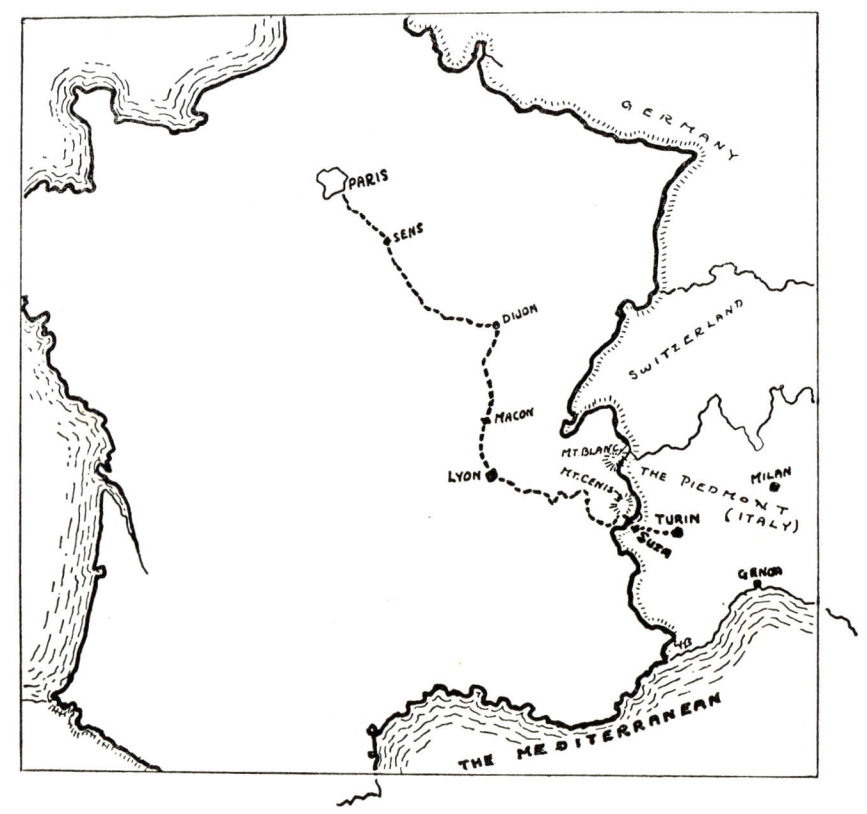

Figure 5. Route of the expedition to Turin (1537-1538).

the fourth edition of his *Oeuvres* dated 1585 (Malgaigne, III, p. 689, and Keynes). Here, again, Paré's date is in error by present calculations; instead of 1536, it should be 1537.

We have read of Paré's part in the battle of the Pass of Suza. The story can continue here.

The defenders of the little castle decided to surrender. They were disarmed and each soldier was given a white staff as a token of his defenselessness. Having no other refuge, most made their way to the Château de Villane, called Avigliana by the Italians, defended by two hundred of the Spaniards. This castle stood on a little mountain where it could not be effectively fired upon by the field artillery. Although it was surrounded by the French, the Marshal could not spare the troops needed to keep it sealed up, nor could he leave it behind, threatening his line of communications. The defenders were called upon to surrender, at the cost of being cut to pieces should an assault be required. They bravely refused, reminding Montmorency that they owed as much allegiance to the Emperor as he did to his King. This left the Marshal no alternative save to capture the castle.

During the night, two huge siege cannon were dragged into position by German and Swiss mercenaries. Unfortunately, a careless gunner fired a couple of bags of gunpowder, by the flash of which he and a dozen other artillerymen were burned. Moreover, the flash betrayed their position, and all through the night the defenders of the castle continued to fire at the spot, killing and wounding a number of the French. Early in the morning, the bombardment started. Within a few hours, a breach was pounded into the walls. The defenders now demanded a parley, but it was too late; Montejan's infantry poured through the breach and cut them to pieces. They did not sell themselves lightly, however. They fought furiousy, killing a great number of the attackers, and wounded so many that the surgeons had heavy work on their hands. Finally, the tumult stilled. The defending captain and an ensign were hanged on the top of the castle gate to warn other Imperialists of the fate in store for those who might thereafter be tempted to hold out against the power of the King's army. All the other living defenders were killed; all but one, as Paré noted. A very pretty young Piedmont girl was spared, as a great Lord wanted her to keep him company in the night, "from fear of the loup-garou" (a legendary were-wolf)!

Now began the work for which Paré had been brought along. The battle surgeons set up crude dressing stations wherever they could, and received the wounded who could walk or be carried to them. They sutured the horribly contused wounds made by swords, battle-axes, and halberds. They lopped off mangled limbs with almost magically swift strokes of their sickle-shaped amputation knives and stanched the spurting arteries by thrusting cherry-red hot cauterizing irons into quivering flesh. Then they puckered the skin down over the oozing stump with several heavy sutures passed with quick thrusts of large needles. Their patients screamed and writhed in the grasp of their restraining friends, or stoically sweated out the pain in dumb silence. More fortunate were those who could faint and regain consciousness later, to suffer only the dull agony of pain for which there was little help except alcohol. To all this, Paré was accustomed through his years of training; only the sudden volume of work was different from the emergencies of the Hôtel-Dieu.

But here he met one new and unfamiliar problem (Hamby, p. 56). Until yesterday, he had had no experience with fresh gunshot wounds. Physicians and surgeons had not yet learned how best to treat this new form of injury, brought to them by the recent introduction of gunpowder into warfare. Paré had read in Jean de Vigo that these wounds were poisoned. It puzzled him that the powder itself was not poisonous; soldiers drank potions of it in water or wine and gave it to their horses and dogs to make them brave and tough. De Vigo had advised treating such wounds by cauterizing them with oil of sambuc or elders, containing a little theriac,[25] applied as hot as possible. Ambroise went to watch the experienced barber-surgeons and learned their technique. They kept the oil in metal pots bubbling in the glowing coals of their braziers where the cauterizing irons were kept at the proper temperature. "Tents" of cotton or linen cloth were dropped into the oil; then, using forceps to protect their fingers, the surgeons lifted the cloth dripping with the boiling oil and thrust it into the depths of the gaping or puckered wounds.

If a wound tract was not open, they probed for the buried bullets, usually a quarter inch or more in diameter. When the probe struck metal, a quick stroke of the razor laid open the wound, through which bloody fingers or pincers removed the ball. The searing oil was applied, the wound was bandaged, and the next casualty was brought up for quick appraisal and treatment. All this Ambroise did, swiftly, deftly and soon almost automatically, as a good surgeon does, releasing his mind to dwell on things more important than mere technique.

Suddenly, the smooth flow of motion was broken. His reaching forceps met no response; his assistant stammered that they had run out of oil. Sorry for the delay, Ambroise quickly reassured the patient and sent the boy to borrow or buy oil from some surgeon who could supply him. He treated patients with other types of wounds until the boy finally returned empty-handed; no more oil was to be had. Here was a fine problem for a green young army surgeon. His youth was enough of a handicap. Now he lacked even proper supplies! Analyzing the situation swiftly, he realized that beyond their "venosity," or being "poisoned," these were essentially penetrating, contused wounds made by large missiles of relatively low velocity, much like arrow wounds. Other such wounds were treated by "digestive" dressings; he could think of nothing better to do with these. His assistant quickly mixed the digestive, of egg yolks, oil of roses, and turpentine, which Paré applied to the wounds before he bandaged them. The patients, no doubt, could hardly believe their good fortune at getting this soothing dressing instead of being blistered and burned as they had seen so often before. Only their young surgeon was tormented with the realization that he had failed them.

This worry did not leave him when Paré finally was able to fall exhausted upon his bed. He spent a restless night and slept little. Finally, giving up the attempt early in the morning, he went to visit his patients, anxious, at least, to know the worst. Then came the happy surprise. Those treated with the simple dressing were not dead of gunpowder poisoning; in fact, they were as well and as comfortable as the size and seriousness of their wounds permitted. Those who had been treated with the customary hot oil, on the other hand, were feverish, with great pain and swelling around their wounds. Not having long-established prejudice to overcome in his own mind, Ambroise realized at once that the hot oil treatment actually was mischievous. Experienced now in the hard life of the soldiers, Paré resolved that henceforth he would do everything possible to prevent them from being subjected to this additional, unnecessary misery. There were no medical journals or surgical meetings then where he could tell his story; he would need to write a book.

At the end of the campaign of conquest of the Piedmont, the French remained as an army of occupation. Paré, staying with them, heard of a local surgeon famous for his success in treating gunshot wounds. Ambroise sought him out and learned that he treated such wounds with a secretly-prepared "balm." He would not share the secret of its preparation, so Ambroise undertook a systematic campaign to obtain it. He made things very agreeable for the Italian surgeon, gave him presents and, no doubt, extended him many courtesies possible for an influential member of a conquering army in occupied territory. Just before leaving the Piedmont forever, Ambroise went to the silent surgeon, begging him to give or sell his secret, since they would not be in competition. The surgeon finally consented. He showed Ambroise how the famous balm was made, warning him not to let the secret get away from him (Malgaigne, II, p. 127). The balm was made by boiling newly whelped puppies in oil of lilies and mixing this stew with earthworms prepared in Venice turpentine! On thinking the matter over, Paré realized that the Italian surgeon's weird mixture was essentially not greatly different from the simpler one he had prepared in his hour of need. The virtue of the dressings lay in avoiding adding fresh injury to the already-damaged tissues. Nevertheless, he faithfully used the Italian's puppy-oil preparation for a number of years.

In December of 1537, the Duke de Montejan was made Governor of the Piedmont. He settled down with a garrison of ten or twelve thousand men scattered through the cities of the area. Paré loved and served the Duke faithfully. He made a fast friend of Montejan's wife, the Duchesse Philippes de Montespedon,[26] who later became godmother of his own son, Ambroise, on 30 May 1576. Since soldiers in garrison do not put aside the belligerent characteristics that made them successful conquerors, they brawled and fought among themselves and the inhabitants. There were many wounds to dress, legs and arms to amputate, and broken heads to trepan. According to Paré's account, he cared for three-fourths of the garrison's accidents, and traveled to other cities of the area to care for patients to whom the Duke sent him.

Once, after a quarrel, two gentlemen began duelling with swords. One gave the other a thrust under the left breast, but the wounded man continued to fight so furiously that his opponent fled. The victim pursued him nearly two hundred yards, then fell dead. Ambroise performed an autopsy and was astonished to find the heart perforated by a wound admitting a fingertip (Malgaigne, II, p. 95; Hamby, p. 49).

Scattered through his *Oeuvres* are references to patients Paré treated in the Piedmont. One day, one of the Marshal's kitchen boys fell into a cauldron of oil almost boiling hot. Going to the apothecaries for the cooling medications usually used in such cases, Ambroise met an old local woman who advised him to treat the scalded lad with onion poultices, since they usually prevented blistering. He asked her if she had really had experience with the method. On being assured that she had, he resolved to try it on this scullion. He covered the burned areas with fresh onions crushed with a little salt, and later he found that where the poultice had touched, no blisters developed (Malgaigne, II, p. 128; Hamby, p. 58).

Some time later (Malgaigne, II, p. 128; Hamby, p. 58), one of the Duke's German mercenaries had his face and hands seriously burned when his powder flask exploded. Ambroise treated the soldier's face with the onion poultice and the other parts with the customary remedies. At the next dressing, the face was free of blisters and excoriations, while the other parts were covered with them. These experiences proved the value of the onion poultice treatment to Paré, and also made him more aware of the value of personal experimentation in seeking new methods better than the old.

Paré was not content to try new medications on hearsay authority alone, but put them to experimental test whenever he could. When arguing a point with an opponent, he used this method of persuasion in preference to quotation of authority, then the major resource of physicians. On one occasion (Malgaigne, II, p. 71; Hamby, p. 39), one of Montejan's pages was struck on the head by a stone thrown by an opponent in a game of quoits. Paré found a compound fracture of the right parietal bone, through which a bit of brain extruded. On this evidence, Paré classed the wound a deadly one. One of the young physicians present argued violently with him, protesting that the extruded tissue was fat and not brain. Ambroise gave him the specimen to hold while he dressed the wound. Then he reminded the young man that the skull does not contain fat, not from Galen's dictum alone, but from his own dissection experience. The physician continued the argument, so Ambroise suggested that the matter be settled by experimentation. Several of the gentlemen and others present wanted to see how this could be done. Ambroise said that if the tissue were fat, it should float on water, and if brain, it should sink. In water, it settled to the bottom of the vessel. To clinch the argument, he put the fragment on a shovel and held it over the fire. Instead of melting into oil, the fragment dessicated and after drying like leather, began to burn. His point proved, Ambroise was fair enough to add to the record that, contrary to his prognosis, the page recovered, although he was permanently deaf.

On another occasion (Malgaigne, II, p. 233; Hamby, p. 74), a common soldier was shot in the wrist by a musket ball that mangled the extremity considerably. The arm, not amputated, soon became infected and gangrenous. The patient became gravely ill, inflammation reaching the elbow and signs of infection extending upward to the chest. Several surgeons who saw the patient declined to treat him because of the gravity of the situation. Finally, the soldier's friends prevailed upon Paré to minister to him. With considerable misgivings, he amputated the arm through the elbow joint, since Hippocrates had said that this could be done without going through the bone. It is noteworthy here that amputations were done at that time only in the distal parts of the extremities; the upper arm and thigh were never removed because of the high mortality from shock and blood loss. Paré stopped the bleeding with cautery, because then he knew no better method. He drained the arm with several incisions made in the stump, and lightly cauterized the exposed end of the humerus. After dressing the arm, Ambroise treated the patient vigorously to restore his strength and to improve his chances for survival. Despite all his attention, the patient developed complications termed convulsions, but which, from the description, seemed to resemble tetanus.

The man was housed in a draughty granary, through the chinks of which the cold wind and the snow blew freely. Paré had him carried to a nearby stable steaming with fresh horse manure. Getting two large braziers to furnish heat, he uncovered the man and massaged his neck and back with liniments considered effective for convulsions. He wrapped the patient in warm linen, had a bed of straw prepared for him in the hot manure, covered him with straw, then buried him to the neck in the manure. After three days, the patient began to sweat; his bowels moved and his jaws relaxed a little. Paré pried them open gently with a screw dilator until he could set a willow stick between the teeth on each side. He then began feeding him raw eggs, milk, and broth. The patient improved gradually. The convulsions ceased. Finally, only the arm remained to be healed—which finally it did. When Ambroise described the case later, he gave God credit for the cure and cautioned young surgeons who read his book not to give up a patient for lost, however desperate his condition appears, "for often such people recover after having been neglected and abandoned."

A Parisian soldier named l'Evesque, under Captain Renouart's command, was wounded with three severe sword thrusts (Malgaigne, II, p. 97; Hamby, p. 51). One entered the chest cavity. The surgeon who first treated him had stitched the wound tightly. The next day the patient had a high fever, and severe pain in his side. He spat blood and could hardly talk. Being called to see him, Paré opened the wound and found it filled with clotted blood.[27] Then he ordered the patient to lie head downward over the edge of the bed, cover up his mouth and nose, and strain to exhale. Blood spurted in a jet from the wound. Paré next put him back in bed and irrigated his chest cavity, washing out more blood clots. The complications diminished, and the man improved. The next day Ambroise again irrigated the wound with a solution containing absinthe and aloes. The patient became nauseated from the bitter solution rising into his mouth, which reminded Paré of a case of tracheobronchial fistula he had seen in the Hôtel-Dieu, and he realized the nature of this wound. Eventually l'Evesque recovered.

A lackey of M. de Goulaines (Malgaigne, II, p. 66; Hamby, p. 37) received a sword stroke of the right parietal region, which did not pierce the inner table of the skull. His wound had almost healed when some of the patient's friends from Gascony visited him. He joined them in feasting and drinking, and in a few days became very ill. He developed a fever, became irrational and unable to talk. His head and face swelled greatly, and his eyes protruded and became inflamed. After examining him, Paré called physicians and surgeons into consultation. The man was bled and given clysters, and his extremities were bandaged. Later, his wound opened and a great deal of pus drained. Finally, an area of the skull as large as the palm of a hand was bared, then became necrotic and infested by maggots. The bone gradually separated and came away; the scalp healed, leaving a large depression. Ambroise had a moulded leather helmet made to protect the man's brain until the scar became very solid and no more protection was needed.

For all his professional ambition, activity, and devotion to duty, Ambroise was a young man of 27 or 28 during his sojourn in Italy. We have no clue as to his extraprofessional activities there. He must have read much, and probably not all his reading was surgical. He later exhibited a flair for rhyming and writing rather amateurish poetry, and his surgical writing certainly developed a forcefulness and charm far removed from the technical jargon of the craftsman narrowly confined to his field.

Associated with the court of the Governor and his Lady, who were important as duke and duchess in their own country; and transported into this softer and more civilized environment at an impressionable age, Ambroise probably absorbed some of the Renaissance influence that was spreading from Italy to France. Even Henri the Dauphin lost some of his dour fierceness there and sired a daughter on a local girl, Filippa Ducci (Williams). This child, called Dianne de France, later was brought to the French Court, educated under the tutelage of Dianne de Poitiers, and married Duke Horace Farnese.

In February of 1538, Governor Montejan received a very high military honor; he was appointed a Marshal of France. Unfortunately, he fell ill with a liver disease, a hepatic flux, as Paré termed it. The Marshal sent to Milan for a famous Italian physician to come to Turin to treat him. Paré may have gone to Milan with the party sent to the physician, or he may have gone there on another occasion. He reported being there, and of learning the method used by a local surgeon for treatment of paraphimosis (Malgaigne, II, p. 554).

The Milanese physician spent some time in Turin with the Marshal, and was called into consultation frequently by the surgeons to see their patients. This physician often took Paré with him and, if the treatment required serious surgery, he saw to it that Paré did it," ". . . which I did promptly and dextrously," Ambroise reported matter-of-factly. The Milanese told Montejan, "You have a surgeon young in years but old in experience and knowledge. Guard him well, for he will give you service and bring you honor." Then Paré added, ". . . but the good man didn't know that I had lived three years in the Hôtel-Dieu de Paris to treat the sick there."

The Marshal's liver got no better, despite the care of the physicians, and in the autumn of 1538 he died. His post fell to Claude d'Annebault, who had commanded the Turin expedition and had earned a Marshal's baton the same year. Ambroise had loved Montejan like a father, and was so desolate at his death that he resolved to return to Paris. The new Governor sought to keep Paré in his service for his reputation had grown so great.

He promised Ambroise to treat him as well as had de Montejan, but when Paré explained his personal grief, the Governor reluctantly let him go. He then returned to Paris, spending eighteen days on the way, and probably traveling by post over the beautiful road he had traversed with the Duke's army two years earlier.

CHAPTER III

The Young Barber-Surgeon in Paris
1538-1542

ALTHOUGH PARE MADE no mention of it that has come down to us, the scene must have shifted so suddenly on his return home that the Piedmont quickly took on the aspects of a dream. He found that his friend de Héry[28] had followed him over the Alps into Italy in 1537. Malgaigne (III, p. xiv) thought that de Héry had gone to Turin with Paré, but he had gone on to Rome to study syphilis in the Hôspital St. Jacques Majori, with a special group sent there for that purpose by François I (Le Paulmier, p. 22). He now was taking courses under Drs. Jacques Houllier[29] and Antoine Saillard. Since the two had been friends together in the service in the Hôtel-Dieu and had worked together for several years, it is unlikely that Ambroise would not have found some reason to mention him in his accounts of that expedition. De Héry has not yet got his license to practice, so he and Ambroise dissected together to sharpen their wits in preparation for their examinations. It seems strange that two such superior candidates should have delayed so long after completing their training before undertaking this formality, which was obligatory. Perhaps they found plenty of interesting work outside independent practice. Perhaps there were unwritten "ground-rules" about which we know nothing. Paré was still accumulating material for the book on anatomy he was writing for the young barber-surgeon apprentices. Under his stimulus, perhaps de Héry even then was beginning to put together his book on syphilis that would appear in 1552.

On invitation, Paré went to see the famous Professor Sylvius,[30] and as he recorded, the visit lasted so long that he remained for dinner. Sylvius was the anatomist under whom Vesalius had come to Paris to study. Because he was a traditional Galenist and no investigator, he disappointed his talented pupil. The two quarreled violently after the appearance of Vesalius' *Fabrica* in 1543. Although Paré never said so, it is likely that he acted as prosector for the Professor in some of the classes for the Medical School and in the Hôtel-Dieu, as was the custom. At any rate, Paré told him of his experiences in the Piedmont, of his treatment of gunshot wounds, of the use of onion poultices for burns, and of a method of more readily findings bullets hidden in the body. Despite his adherence to the traditions of the Faculté in its relations to the barber-surgeons and its opposition to medical writings in the vernacular, "the good old man" urged Paré to write up these discoveries, particularly to overcome the effects of Jean de Vigo's teachings on the treatment of gunshot wounds. (Malgaigne, II, p. 128). The response of the young surgeon to this encouragement can well be imagined.

At the end of 1540, Paré and de Héry took the first examinations for their licenses. Early in 1541, they took the second, paid the fee of "72 sols 6 deniers Paresis," made their vows at the church of St. Sépulchre in rue St. Denis to support the Corporation of Barber-surgeons, and so became Master Barber-surgeons. The first major hurdle on the way to legitimate practice lay behind them. Malgaigne was not familiar with these details; it remained for Le Paulmier to unearth the records (p. 22).

Ambroise probably was quite busy then, establishing a practice of his own. He had been back in Paris from Italy for almost two years, and in June of 1541, he took another step common for the young surgeon starting practice; he got married.

Regretably, we have no record of how Ambroise met his fiancee. Jeanne Mazelin[31] was the 20-year-old niece of Méry de Prime, a wine-seller whose shop faced the Place St. Michel at the corner of the rue de l'Hirondelle. Her step-father, Étienne Cléret, was a shop-keeper in the rue St. André-des-Arts. This was the neighborhood in which Ambroise had lived since coming to Paris. Jeanne's father, Jean Mazelin, had been a clerk of Cardinal DuPrat, who had built the new ward at the Hôtel-Dieu just before Paré went there. Her father probably shared the disgrace of his chief, and he had died earlier. His wife and Jeanne's mother, Jeanne de Prime, was a sister of Méry de Prime. After Mazelin's death, she had married Étienne Cléret, the merchant of rue St. André-des-Arts.

On 30 June 1541, Ambroise and Jeanne went before Jean Dupré and Remon d'Orléans, notaries at the Châtelet, and signed the marriage contract (Le Paulmier, p. 143). Witnesses included Jeanne's uncle Méry and her aunt Marguerite Choisel, widow of the late Odo de Prime, Méry's brother, who had been a Master Barber-surgeon. Paré's witnesses were Étienne de la Rivière[32] and Loys Drouet,[33] also Master Barber-surgeons. Jeanne's dowry was six hundred livres tournois. The other details were reported by Le Paulmier, and were unknown to Malgaigne. The six hundred livres were paid the young couple on 16 July and they were married a few days later, for in a receipt for the money, Jeanne was called Ambroise's fiancee and not his wife. They were married in St. André-des-Arts, the parish church that remained his religious center through the rest of Ambroise's life.

Paré's witness, Rivière, was an important man who remained his friend as long as he lived. In association with the physician, Charles Estienne,[34] he had been engaged in dissecting and drawing illustrations for the most ambitious Anatomy that had been projected before that of Vesalius. Estienne was a member of a famous family of printers, which gave him unusual entre into book production. Among the illustrations for the book were drawings made by Rivière and another group of pictures of rather tortured-looking subjects displaying their viscera. Kellett quoted Singer and Rabin's remark that "this book of Estienne's is the ugliest of anatomical studies we know." Only recently has Dr. Kellett shown that these illustrations were printed from art blocks owned by the publishing house, modified by inserts into anatomical illustrations. When the time came for publication, Estienne proposed to publish the book under his name alone, ignoring Rivière completely, as would a physician of the time. Rivière promptly stopped the presses by entering suit before Parlement. The trial dragged out for several years and finally judgement was rendered in Rivière's favor, in this same year. He will return to our attention repeatedly hereafter.

We do not know where Ambroise and Jeanne lived in the early years of their marriage. They had a number of relatives on each side of the family living around the Place St. Michel, and they may have lived with one of them. Ambroise would have needed a shop for his barbering, for he probably followed the customs of his time by keeping his shop open all day. He was busy also in the dissecting room and at the Medical School, because he wrote as if he never interrupted that enterprise, so he must have needed someone to assist him. Even in his Turin days he wrote of "my man" who helped him in his duties. He acquired apprentices who lived in his home, but we do not know when this developed.

In 1542, France, Sweden and Denmark declared war upon the Emperor, Charles V. While battles raged in the north of France, at the other end of the country, an attempt was being made to dislodge the Spaniards from Perpignan. This town, on the Spanish border roughly fifteen kilometers from the Gulf of Lyon, stands in the foothills of the Pyrennes on the south shore of the river Têt. The Duke d'Annebault, with forty thousand men, came down from the Piedmont to besiege the place. When the Vicount de Rohan[35] was ordered to Perpignan, he called Paré to join him. Although this was his second military expedition as a surgeon, it was the first to interrupt Paré's practice and to take him from his bride. This, of course, was to become the pattern of his life. Ambroise rode with de Rohan to Perpignan by post, changing horses often enough to permit the desired speed of transit within their range of endurance. They must have ridden fast in the late August (1542) heat for, when they reached Lyon, half-way to their destination, Ambroise suffered an attack of hematuria. He must have recovered rapidly, since when he mentioned the incident later (Malgaigne, II, p. 500; Hamby, p. 93), he gave no indication of ever having suffered another. Although he said nothing of it, Ambroise must a also have been delighted with and interested in the beauties of Provence, as is every first visitor to the area.

In his *Journeys*, Ambroise described two cases he had treated in the camp (Malgaigne, III, p. 694; Hamby, p. 165). On one occasion, the Spaniards made a sally from the town and overran

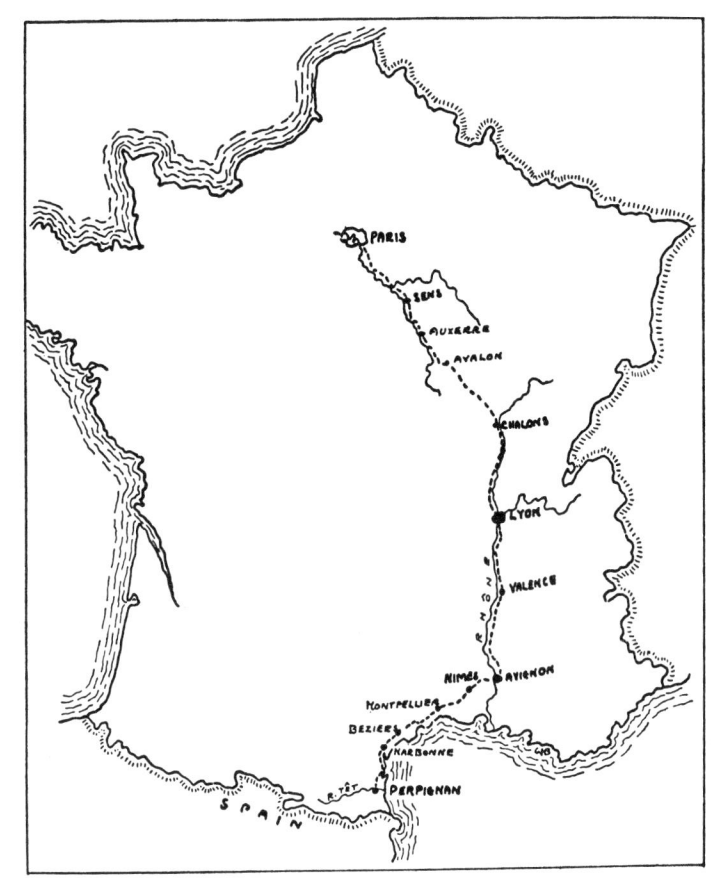

Figure 6. Route of the expedition to Perpignan (1542).

a French artillery position. The Grand-Master of Artillery himself, the Count de Brissac,[36] happened to be there. The Spaniards, beaten off, regained the protection of the walls, but not without killing and wounding a number of the French. De Brissac himself was shot in the shoulder. As he returned to his tent, the other wounded followed him, hoping to be dressed by the surgeons attending their Chief.

The Count got to bed and the surgeons got to work. Three or four of the most expert of the army tried unsuccessfully to locate the bullet with their probes. Baffled, they reasoned that since no wound of exit was found, it must have glanced off into the body. Having known Paré from the Piedmont campaign, de Brissac sent for him to see what he could do. Realizing that this was an unusual case, since the obvious had failed, Ambroise asked the Count to get out of bed and to assume the position in which he had been when shot. Taking a javelin in his hands, the Count crouched into position. Ambroise ran his hand over the Count's back. There, under the muscles around the shoulder blade, he felt the swelling made by the ball. The thirty-two-year old Paré then made a characteristic gesture. Having found the ball, he did not monopolize the spotlight; he gracefully declined the privilege of removing the missile. The Dauphin's surgeon, M. Nicole Lavernault, performed the operation on the Count. It probably was no mere coincidence that M. Lavernault, later Surgeon of King François, then of Henri II and finally Premier-surgeon of Charles IX, remained Paré's friend. He was an official of the College of St. Côme when Paré was admitted to membership in 1554. When Lavernault died in 1561, Paré succeeded him as Premier-surgeon of King Charles IX.

Paré reported a case that amazed him at Perpignan (Malgaigne III, p. 695; Hamby, p. 165). In his presence, a soldier struck with his halberd a fellow soldier who was cheating at dice. Although the heavy war axe sliced through the fellow's skull and into the left lateral ventricle of the brain, he did not even fall. Amazed that the man had not died instantly, Paré dressed him at the insistence of some of his friends, and incredulously watched him stagger along to his lodgings some two hundred yards away. He advised a friend of the wounded man to get a priest for him, since he would surely die. The next day Paré was visited by the soldier's girl companion, dressed as a boy, who implored him to come and dress her protector's wound. Fearing that the man would die under his hands, Paré put her off with the remark that the dressing should not be disturbed for three days. Surely this, he thought, should be time enough for nature to take its course. On the third day, however, into his tent staggered the hapless man and his wench. He begged Ambroise to dress his head, and promised to pay his fee, showing him a purse holding a hundred or more gold pieces. Again, the surgeon tried to evade removing the dressing; finally, at the insistence of some Gentlemen who had become interested in the case, he reluctantly consented. His worst fears were soon realized; when the dressing was removed, the patient had a convulsion and died. The priest, who had remained with the man throughout his ordeal, now attached his purse, "to say masses for his soul," and to see that no one else got it. In addition, he got away with the dead man's clothes and other property—no mention was made of the disposition of the girl—leaving Ambroise to marvel that, with his brain split, the man had retained his senses to the moment of his death, three days later.

Soon afterward, the fortunes of the attackers declined. Information arrived that four companies of Spaniards had fought their way into the city to reinforce the defense. Plague struck the French camp. The local people warned the soldiers that the rising winds from the sea would flood their camp, laid out in the river valley. The prediction was quickly verified. The wind became a great storm that scourged the area. A race was begun to break camp. Before it could be accomplished, however, many carts with their drivers and draft mules were swept away in the flood. A great deal of baggage was lost. Ambroise informed us quite noncommittally that he then returned to Paris.

The dates that Paré gave for some of his army experiences have been found erroneous. Indeed, he himself said later that he did not have the dates well in mind while writing the accounts, but that the stories and reports all were accurate. He indicated that he went to Picardy first, then to Landrecies, then to Perpignan and to Boulogne. Le Paulmier (p. 24) found a somewhat different sequence from official documents. His corrected itinerary will be followed here.

In 1543, François and the Dauphin invaded Heinault[37] with thirty-five thousand men and encamped at Maroilles, a village ten kilometers from Avesnes, near the present Belgian border. In June, de Rohan took Paré there as his surgeon (Malgiagne, III, p. 692). Before they could see action, word came from the Duke d'Estampes,[38] Governor of Brittany, that the English had sailed to attack Low-Brittany. He asked the King to send the Duke de Laval[39] and the Vicount de Rohan to help command the defense. These Lords were of that part of the country and

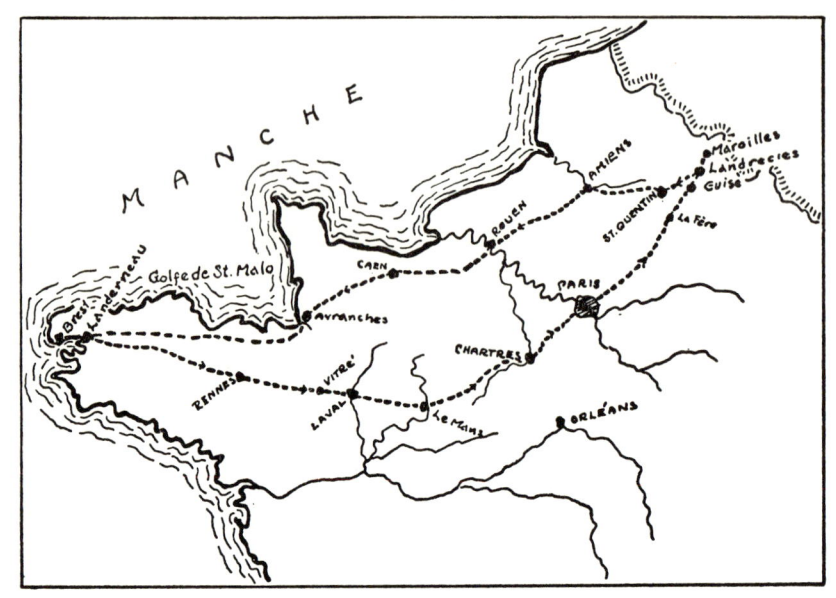

Figure 7. Route of the expedition to Maroilles and Landerneau (1543).

the local people would fight under them more effectively than under strangers.

The King was under personal obligation to d'Estampes, who had married François' mistress, Anne de Pisseleau, to give her a place at the Court, if not to make her an honest woman, exactly. The two requested officers were dispatched immediately; they took Paré and his man with them. Traveling by post again, the party rode, in a week, to Landerneau, near Brest at the tip of Brittany, a distance of about four hundred miles.

In the account recorded in his *Journeys,* Ambroise described the situation in some detail. They found the people in arms. Alarm bells were ringing around all the harbors near Brest, Le Conquet, Crozon, La Fou, Doulac and Laudanec. Well supplied with artillery, all were resolved to prevent an enemy landing. The English sailed in. Uncovering their guns, the French poured a murderous fire into the fleet. Ambroise marvelled to see the cannon balls from the big guns bound and skip over the water as they did on the ground. A landing being impossible, the English ships hoisted sail, and, in good order, took to sea again:

"like a forest marching on the sea." Paré was grateful that the English got away without much injury to themselves or to the French.

The commanders decided to remain there in garrison for a while, to be sure another invasion would not be attempted. Ambroise described interesting details of garrison life of the time. Tournaments were held for the knights; horse races and maneuvers were organized. The Duke d'Estampes had Brittany girls brought into the camp to sing in their dialect, which to Paré sounded like "the singing of frogs in love." They danced the Brittany triary, which "was done with greet agitation of the feet and buttocks." Dancing, duels and wrestling matches provided enough injuries to keep the surgeons busy. Wrestling matches, in which the local champions competed for prizes, seldom ended without a broken arm or leg.

Ambroise described a bout between a huge school master named Dativo and a little squat Breton who had thrown several contestants. Although they looked ridiculously mismatched, the little man threw the giant school teacher sprawling. In a rage, he grappled for another turn and soon contrived to fall unfairly upon the smaller man in such a way as to kill him. Ambroise then did an autopsy; he found a massive thoracic and abdominal hemorrhage, the source of which escaped him, although he searched for it carefully (Malgaigne, III, p. 693; Hamby, p. 163).

Tiring of this garrison life rather quickly probably, although it was routine for the soldiers, Paré got permission to leave. He must have satisfied his superiors, for they gave him rich presents to take with him. M. de Rohan gave him fifty "double ducats" and a hackney horse to ride; M. de Laval gave him a horse for his man; M. d'Estampes gave him a diamond worth thirty crowns,—"and so I returned to my house in Paris."

From Landerneau to Paris, one may go along the north Brittany coast via Rouen, but the more direct route is by way of Rennes, Laval, Le Mans and Chartres. Although he didn't tell us so, his obvious affection for his friends and family probably caused Ambroise to take the latter route and stop at Laval for a visit with those he had left twelve years earlier as a poor barber-surgeon's apprentice.

On his return to the City, Paré found that Vesalius' *Fabrica* had been published. Although he could not read its Latin text, he must have thrilled at its incomparable wood-cuts of anatomy, absorbed in his own version as he was. One could always hire some poor Doctor of the Faculté to translate the Latin!

After Ambroise left the King at Maroilles, the army had not been idle. A detachment under the Duke de Cleves[40] had to surrender to the Emperor on September 7. This so annoyed the King that he annulled the Duke's marriage to his niece, Jeanne d'Albret. On September 10, Luxembourg again fell to the French. In October, Paré went to Landrecies to join the French army. He described it as of 1544, but Le Paulmier, p. 24, corrected the date. The army came face to face with an even larger Imperial force, and Ambroise was surprised that the two great forces did not join in a decisive battle. They confined their action to skirmishes and personal fights, which gave the surgeons plenty of work to do. François was content to supply Landrecies and to withdraw to Guise. Paré returned to Paris, where his first book was in press.

Fifteen hundred-forty-five was an eventful year for the Parés; their first son was born, Ambroise's first book was published, and their friend de la Rivière finally saw his illustrations appear with the anatomy text of Charles Estienne. After de la Rivière won his suit in Parlement, the College of Surgeons of St. Côme admitted the barber-surgeon to its ranks. When the book appeared, he was listed as a surgeon. It was a handsomely produced book, worthy of the great press of Estienne's father-in-law, Simon de Colines. It was entitled, *De Dissectione Partium Corporis Humani Libre Tres, a Carolo Stephano, doctore Medico, Editi. Una cum figuris, & incisionem declarationibus, a Stephano Rivero Chirurgo compositis.* Unfortunately, the legal delay permitted Vesalius to steal a march on the two Frenchmen. Unfortunately too, the almost five years delay also permitted pirating of some of its already printed illustrations, which turned up in various places prior to the official publication, leaving a teasing puzzle for future historians: who plagiarized whom? Cushing (pp. 32-40) considered this problem in considerable detail. Paré must have been happy for his friend, who had not only helped write such a book, but had succeeded in crossing the line drawn so sharply between the lowly barber-surgeons and the haughty surgeons of the Long Red Robe.

In August, 1545, appeared Paré's own book, *La Methode de Traicter Les Playes Faictes Par Hacquebutes Et Autres bastions a feu,* etc.—*Composee par Ambroyse Paré maistre Barbier, Chirurgien à Paris* (The Method of Treating Wounds made by Harquebuses and other Fire-Arms—). It contained 64 text pages with 23 wood-cut illustrations. The little book was published by Vivant Gualterot, whose shop was on the rue St. Jacques, near Paré's home. It was a modest volume, inexpensively printed and bound for the hard use he anticipated for it as a handbook for the battlefields. This has been called "the first scientific book written in French," but Doe remarked that in the British Museum are at least thirty earlier French scientific titles, of which several are medical. Paré's book, however, has the distinction of being the first French treatise concerning treatment of the relatively new gunshot wounds with which the barber-surgeons had to cope. It was written for their instruction, and it made Paré famous. In his preface "To Young Surgeons of Good Will," he hoped that they would find it useful and promised to write more if they did. He said that he had been inspired by Sylvius' encouragement and attributed any good he did to the glory of God. It was dedicated to his friend and Chief-at-Arms, "The Very Illustrious and Very Powerful Lord, Monseigneur Réné, Viconte de Rohan."

On 4 July, 1545, the Paré's first child, François, was baptized at St. André-des-Arts church. Le Paulmier found this record; misled by Bégin's data, and unacquainted with this, Malgaigne (Intro., cccii) knew of no children by Jeanne Mazelin, and of only two daughters by Ambroise's second wife. Little François had as godfathers the physician François de Villenueve and Loys Drouet, the barber-surgeon who had stood up for Ambroise at his wedding. The godmother was the infant's grandmother, Jeanne de Prime. This little fellow was fated to die within a few months and no more children would brighten the Paré household for fourteen years.

CHAPTER IV

The Development of the Military Surgeon
1542-1552

BOULOGNE

Hardly had M. De Rohan received his copy of Paré's book before they were off to the wars again, this time to Boulogne to keep the English from feeling neglected. Ambroise tells (Malgaigne, III, p. 696) how the English came out of their forts to fight in the open.

One day while Ambroise was going through the camp to dress his patients, the English fired a cannon from a tower at a pair of horsemen who had paused to talk. One of them fell to the ground and was believed to have been struck. On examination it was found that the ball had not touched him; his thigh had been severely bruised, apparently by the mere passage of the missile. Paré incised the thigh to drain the contusion. After wounding the horsemen, the ball bounded over the ground and killed four other soldiers. Ambroise was near enough to feel the air-blast himself and he confessed to ducking his own head. The soldiers teased him for being afraid, but he remarked to "my little master," as he addressed Gourmelen,[41] to whom the *Journeys* was addressed, that had he been there, he would not have been afraid **alone!**

Here Paré also described the famous wound of François de Lorraine,[42] later to be Duke de Guise. This history was published again in the second edition of the *Gunshot Wounds* in 1552 (Malgaigne, II, p. 25; Hamby, p. 27). The twenty-six year old knight, already a famous warrior, was accustomed to riding into a charge with the visor of his helmet open. A lance caught him above the right eye, coursed downward through the nose and out the left side of the face between the neck and the ear. The lance shaft was broken off, leaving the metal head imbedded in the wound so solidly that it had to be pulled out by brute force with blacksmith's tongs, the surgeon resting his foot on the knight's forehead. Paget (p. 126) reported an account by a surgeon of M. de Châtillon, later to be the great Coligny,[43] who wrote in some detail of how Paré removed the lance head and treated the wound. Although this makes interesting reading, it probably is untrue. In his accounts, Paré gave many case histories and he carefully differentiated between the patients he treated and those treated by others. Nowhere does he take credit for this remarkable cure. Since the Duke later became an honored friend of his, he certainly would have done so. He simply attributed the Duke's recovery to the grace of God, the recourse of good surgeons. François de Guise thereafter was known familiarly as the "Balafré," or "Scarface," as modern Americans would say.

After the Boulogne campaign, Paré returned to Paris where he lived, practiced and wrote for another five years before going off to the wars again, and again it would be to Boulogne.

Considering the duration and the effects of the lawsuit between Charles Estienne and Étienne de la Rivière over the authorship of their *Anatomy,* the two men would hardly have been expected to remain friends. It is interesting to find that only a year after the publication of the Latin edition of their book, the authors collaborated in the publication of a French edition. This was entitled: *La Dissection des Parties du Corps Humain—divisée en trois livres, faictz par Charles Estienne docteur en Medecine: avec les figures & declaratio des incisiones, composées par Estienne de la Rivière Chirurgien.* Also published by Simon de Colines, this book was as pretentious as the Latin edition had been, although the paper was not quite so good. While this *Anatomy* was in the vernacular, its cost put it beyond the reach of the barber-surgeon apprentices who so badly needed such a text, and its size, 36 x 24 cm, made it too bulky to be carried easily to the battlefields or on rounds by the busy surgeon. With Thierry de Héry and Jean Colombier, Ambroise continued his dissections and his writing to fill that need.

On 28 January, 1547, Henry VIII died in England. He and François had been friendly in their youth, but had been divided by tensions produced by Charles V and had spent practically all their lives fighting. Yet, when François heard of his death, he suddenly felt the premonition of his own end. The magnificent Renaissance King felt his age; he was fifty-four, and a disillusioned old man. He had lived contemptuously with his syphilis for years, but now it took its toll. His favorite sons were dead, and the survivor, Henri, was coldly indifferent to him. After one more rebellious, over-extended hunting expedition, he died at Rambouillet on 31 March, 1547.

Designated his father's heir, Henri II lost no time in taking over the reins of the kingdom. François' favorites were displaced from their posts and were replaced by his own friends: Montmorency was recalled and made Chief of the Privy Council. Antoine de Bourbon,[44] later the King of Navarre, M. de St. André,[45] and the three Guises, François, Charles,[46] Cardinal de Guise, and Louis[47] were taken into the Royal Council. On 26 July, 1547, Henri was crowned at Reims and later Catherine de' Médicis was crowned Queen.

In 1547 also, Paré's book on *Gunshot Wounds* was translated into the Dutch and was published in Antwerp by Jan Roelants: *Een suuerlick Tractact om Corte to handlen ende to genesen alderhande won den en quetsuren ghedaen met haeckbusen—* etc., with 36 woodcuts after the French originals. Thus Paré's little handbook became known to army surgeons beyond the frontiers. Guillemeau later said that such translations had been made also into Spanish and Italian, but this is the only one in a foreign language that Doe was able to find.

In this year also, Dr. Philippe de Flexelles[48] published an *Introduction pour parvenir a la vraye conaissance de la chirurgie raisonelle*. Malgaigne regretfully concluded that Paré had shamelessly plagiarized from this book, but Doe (p. 23) believed that he had merely used it as a syllabus for the Introduction to his *Oeuvres*. At any rate, Ambroise and Dr. Flexelles were friends, for Ambroise reported (Malgaigne, III, p. 50; Hamby, p. 120) going to his house, although he did not date the visit.

Together they went to Champigny, two leagues from Paris, where the Doctor had a little house. Walking in the courtyard, they were accosted by a "big, robust trollop" asking alms. Lifting her skirts, she displayed a piece of bowel hanging down six inches or more. It leaked purulent looking fluid that had fouled her thighs and chemise, a most repulsive sight. The Doctor asked her how long she had suffered from this ailment, and she told him about four years. He quickly noted her robust, "plump-buttocked" status against the lesion. Immediately he jumped upon her, kicking and pummeling her until the object fell to the ground, squirting its contents. It proved to be a beef-bowel filled with blood and milk, tied at each end and punctured at intervals to let the liquid escape slowly. The woman fell to the ground, feigning death. The Doctor ran to the house, apparently to call the gendarmes. Seeing the gate open, the woman took off running and "was never again seen in Champigny."

On the first of January, it was customary for the king to reappoint his medical and surgical staffs. In 1548, the post of Premier-Physician was offered to the famous Dr. Jean Fernel. Due to the press of duties, he requested permission to refuse the honor and asked that it be given instead to Dr. Louis de Bourges,[49] who had been Physician-in-Ordinary under King François since 1527. Henri acted accordingly.

Paré's *Anatomy*, on which he had worked for so long, was ready for the printer and on 6 June, 1549, he was granted for five years the Royal Privilege of printing it. *The Briefve Collection de L'Administration Anatomique: avec la maniere de coioindre les os: Et d'extraire les infants tât mors que vivans du ventre de la mere*—etc. *Corposée par Ambroise Paré maistre Barbier Chyrurgien à Paris*; published by Guillaume Cavellat, at the sign of the Fat Hen in front of the College de Cambrai.

This was the inexpensive anatomy, written for the barber-surgeons' apprentices. It was a pocket-sized book containing 96 pages, no illustrations. It was dedicated, as his last had been, to his friend and employer at the wars, Réné, Viconte de Rohan.

Lacking an academic background, Ambroise had required a frame upon which to model his own production. As he acknowledged, he found this in the French translation by Jean Canappe of the *Anatomical Tables* of Loys Vassé. Vassé, a student of Sylvius, in 1540 had published an abridged anatomy taken from Galen, entitled *In anatomen corporis humain tabulae quatuor*. Vassé followed a plan unusual for the ancients, and more like that of the Italian anatomists. Vassé's 1543 edition was printed by Vivant Gaulterot, who in 1545 had printed Paré's first book on *Gunshot Wounds*. In 1542, appeared Jean Canappe's translation of Vassé, *Tables Anatomiques du Corps Humain soit de l'homme ou de la femme, premierement composees en latin par maistre Loys Vasse, et depuis traduites en francoys par maistre Jean Canappe* (*Anatomic Tables of the Human Body, both male and female*, first composed in Latin by Master Loys Vassé and translated into French by Master Jean Canappe, Lyon, Étienne Dolet,[49] 1542). Chauvelot remarked that the *Briefve Collection* is a sort of Parisian edition of Vassé-Canappe's *Tables*, which are a resume of Galen. It is more than that, however; it was written for an uneducated audience by a man cognizant of their needs, and who so well performed his task that practically all the copies have been worn out in use (Cushing, p. 90).

In the last few pages was included a description of podalic version. This was not original with Paré, as had been widely supposed later. Doe (p. 45) called it the first description of the procedure published since the ancients. Paré said that he had watched the maneuver performed by Thierry de Héry and by Nicole Lambert.[50] This section again has been the subject for discussion of plagiarism most recently by Chauvelot (1958). He concluded that Malgaigne was correct; podalic version was a Middle Ages discovery by unknowns, commonly practiced by Parisian barber-surgeons.

In this book is Paré's lament that he had not had the opportunity to learn Greek and Latin in his youth, and again he promised to write more if this were well received. It must have been, and must have found a ready market, for a year later it was necessary to put out a reprint.

In August of 1549, according to Le Paulmier, p. 29, Bertrand Paré came to Paris from Vitré to live with Ambroise and Jeanne. He was the son of Ambroise's barber-surgeon brother, who had died an unrecorded time earlier. The Parés had no living children and apparently intended to raise the boy as their son. They went to their lawyers, Dupré and d'Orleans, at the Châtelet on August 5 and made a bequest of forty livres tournois annually to the boy in the event of their deaths, should they remain childless. On 20 August, they reappeared with the lad before the attorneys and made the legal bequest, appointing M. Nicole Ezelin, notary to the Châtelet, as Bertrand's trustee. Paré enrolled Bertrand as a student at the College of Surgeons of the Confraternity of St. Côme, intending to bring him up as an educated surgeon. Either the boy was lazy or could not learn, so Ambroise withdrew him from the school and apprenticed him to an apothecary, Jean de St. Germain. Apparently, Bertrand could not learn drugs any better than he could surgery, so he fled that job also. He simply disappeared from the record; no more is known of him.

Later in the same year, Ambroise's other brother, Jean, lost his wife, Marie Périer. This brother was the trunk-maker whose shop was on the rue de la Huchette, east of the Place St. Michel, in the neighborhood where Ambroise and Jean lived. A few months later, three relatives of Marie Périer legally ceded to Jean Paré their rights of succession to her property (Le Paulmier, pp. 163, 166 & 169). These were Jean Naquier, Master Spur-Maker, and his wife Catherine Périer; Jean Mignon, Master Painter and his wife Barbe Périer; and François Périer, also a Master Painter. Ambroise appreciated and remembered the kindness of the Périers to his brother and reciprocated in 1562, when he deeded a part of his property to them to build a house behind his own, facing the Seine (Le Paulmier, p. 59).

BOULOGNE

On 24 April, 1550, the French reoccupied Boulogne and Paré returned there, probably with de Rohan again. While he was there, the second edition of his 1549 *Anatomy* came off the press. It contained a number of uncorrected typographical errors for which Paré apologized. On a page that had been blank in the first ediiton was a *Notice to the Reader* in which the author explained that the book had been printed while he was at camp at Boulogne, so errors beyond his control had crept in. He requested that readers correct these in their copies. This edition also was dedicated to de Rohan.

Another famous book appeared this year, the *Odes* of Pierre de Ronsard (1524-1585). The young poet was one of the seven who took the name of the Pléiade, having the aim of rejuvenating and standardizing the French language. Ronsard later became a favorite of the Court of Charles IX and was called "The Prince of Poets." He and Paré became such friends that a poem of his, dedicated to Paré, was published in all the editions of his *Oeuvres*. Apparently, he even influenced Ambroise to try his hand at the gentle art, for numerous examples of Paré's verse are scattered thru his own and his friends publications.

On 9 September, 1550, Ambroise again went to the law (Le Paulmier, p. 32). His brother-in-law, Antoine Mazelin was a chancellory clerk of the Court, living at Tours. Apparently his expenses were greater than his income, for, on 31 March 1546, he had borrowed 40 écus of gold, approximately $150, from Ambroise. The loan was secured by shares of his patrimony. Now Ambroise and three other creditor members of the Mazelin family foreclosed on Antoine. The transaction must have been a friendly family affair, for nine years later Antoine, still a Court clerk, stood godfather for Ambroise's son Isaac.

In this deal, Ambroise became a quarter-share owner of property, with his wife Jeanne; with Catherine de Prime, wife of Pierre de la Rue, a tailor who lived nearby; and the wife of Charles Fournier, another of Jeanne's relatives. The property consisted of a Parisian house known, from the sign of a cow hanging on it, as the Maison de la Vache. It was in the rue de l'Hirondelle, next door to the wineshop of Jeanne's uncle Méry de Prime. On the other side was a house carrying the sign of the Three Moors, the Maison des Trois Maures, belonging to Jean Mastreau. The Maison de la Vache had living rooms, cellar, a basement room, upper rooms and an attic; in the rear courtyard were two out-houses. The house was roofed with tiles. The Parés moved into the Maison de la Vache and lived there until sometime before 1561, when Ambroise bought the Maison des Trois Maures, in which he spent the rest of his life. He eventually owned a large part of the end of the block between the Place St. Michel, the Quai-des-Grands-Augustins and the rue de l'Hirondelle.

This area was mapped by Le Paulmier, p. 172, unfortunately from an undisclosed source, and the map was reproduced by Paget, p. 177. It is not included here, since the houses of the area no longer exist, as was true, indeed, in Paget's day. In the larger house, Paré had room for growth. He needed room for his shop and his apprentices, and probably for a study in which he could keep his books and his expanding literary materials. By now, he had several books in progress. He started a museum of his curiosities of medical and natural historical material. Obtaining the corpse of a hanged criminal from the authorities, he dissected half of it completely so he could more readily refresh his memory about obscure anatomical points. His description of this preparation can be found in Malgaigne, III, p. 673.

It is difficult now to precisely identify the sites of the Paré property, for the area was reconstructed in the mid-19th century. St. Michel's Bridge was replaced in 1857 by the present one, built down-river a bit from the original, which then was removed (Clunn, p. 86). The Place St. Michel, enlarged greatly, now engulfs the area where the Paré houses stood.

In addition to the Maison de la Vache, Paré also got part ownership of a house and several plots of vineyard in the village of Meudon, about six miles from the city property. The house, on the rue des Pierres, also was described by Le Paulmier, p. 173, from legal records. It was divided, one part behind the other, with a court and a small garden between them. The court contained a tile-roofed outhouse and a well. Behind the house was a garden with trees and a grape-arbor. The vineyards consisted of eleven scattered plots ranging in size from one-eighth to one and a half acres, totaling about five acres. Ownership of each of these eleven plots was divided among two to four people or estates, making it a very complicated affair. It seems that Paré eventually bought out at least some of the other shareholders. The plots were near the cemetery and the present railway station and have not been identified, as far as I know.

Paré apparently disposed of the Meudon property during his lifetime; it did not appear in his will.

Le Paulmier (p. 174) attempted to locate the Meudon house. It was on the rue des Pierres, "behind the church," he said. Such a description has little meaning now; the street is a good hundred yards up the hill from the church, and the intervening space is built up solidly with houses. Le Paulmier located the house at #9, in his own lifetime next door to #11, belonging in 1676 to Armande Bejart, widow of Moliere. At present, this place is the town museum and is said to have been preserved in its original form. Its only inclusion of its famous neighbor is a small framed steel-engraved portrait; the museum attendants knew nothing of Ambroise Paré. In 1957, the house at #9 was found torn down, its tiles piled neatly along the curb of the narrow, cobble-stoned street. The plot was roughly fifty by one hundred and fifty feet in extent, and probably was the one to which Le Paulmier referred.

Meudon is approximately six miles from the site of Paré's town houses. To reach it, he rode horseback over the rue St. André-des-Arts, through the Port de Bucy, past St. Germain-des-Prés and out into the country southwestward along the route of the present rue de Sevres. He could make the journey in less than an hour. It is almost impossible to do it in less time now by automobile through the traffic and the one-way streets, especially if one wanders inadvertently into the Citröen factory area that stretches along the riverside. If one climbs the crooked, narrow little rue des Pierres to the top of the steep hill, he finds a splendid Terrasse, approximately a half-mile long, from which there is a perfectly beautiful view across Paris to the church of Sacre-Coeur on Montmartre. Here, François I built a château for his mistress, the Duchesse d'Estampes. Diane de Poitiers took it over after François' death and later sold it to the Cardinal de Lorraine, who enlarged it grandly. It reverted to and was kept in the royal family by Louis XIV for Monseigneur, his only legitimate son to survive childhood. After Monseigneur and his children died there of smallpox in 1711 the château passed to Louis XV and XVI, who used it as a stopping place on the way to Versailles. During the Revolution, it was used as an arsenal and was partly demolished by a powder explosion. In 1871, the Germans put a gun emplacement on the Terrasse to bear on the city.

On 18 January, 1551, Rabelais (1490-1553) was made Curé of Meudon, and his status now stands before the Mairie. Although this famous writer was a priest and a physician, graduated from Montpellier in 1537, neither he nor Paré mentioned the other in his writings. Rabelais died two years after his appointment; it is unlikely that he ever actually served the parish personally. It was common practice then for the income from the parish of such a church to be given to support clerics attached to the Court.

Paré had obtained the Royal Privilege of reprinting his 1545 book on *Gunshot Wounds* on 4 February 1551. This was an enlarged version of the first, containing forty-three woodcut illustrations (Doe p. 29), including pictures of artificial limbs. Paré had had these illustrations cut after long negotiations with the makers of the appliances, indicating that there were specialists in the craft even then.

On the advice of the Viconte de Rohan, this volume was to be dedicated to the King, so Paré had it printed by a new publisher who could do a more artistic job than could Gaulterot; this was Agnes Sucevin, the widow of Jean de Brie. Her publishing house was a successful one, although various of its members were in trouble intermittently for publishing Huguenot literature. She did a beautiful job, and three vellum copies were made for presentation to Royalty. One of these was given to Diane de Poitiers. Its rich bindings were stamped with her device: H-for-Henri, intertwined with Cs, ostensibly for Catherine, but so contrived that the tips of the crescents touched the uprights of the H to make Ds, for Diane. The printing of this book was completed on 10 March, 1552.

A week later the army was called out suddenly, to assemble at Châlons-sur-Marne, forty thousand strong. Henri and the Emperor had come to a definitive test of arms. The French army was under the command of the Constable Montmorency. The Constable's nephew, Gaspard de Châtillon, Duke de Coligny, was chief Colonel of Infantry, with twenty thousand landsquenets,[51] two regiments of each captained by M. Record and M. Ringrave.[52] Captain Châstel led the troops provided by the allied Protestant Princes. Claude de Guise, Duke d'Aumale, younger brother of François de Guise, was General of Cavalry. This force consisted of five hundred knights, who with retainers numbered forty-five hundred mounted men; two thousand Light Horse and two thousand mounted arquebusiers. The King was accompanied by two hundred Gentlemen of his Household (with their numerous retainers) under the Sieur de Boisy, and his escort contained six hundred French, Scottish and Swiss Guards, with four hundred lances commanded by the Dauphin, the Duke de Guise, the Duke d'Aumale and the Marshal St. André. Paré (Malgaigne, III, p. 697) described the sight as a thing marvelous to see; indeed it must have been as the long, colorful procession filled the roads leading eastward. Paré went along again as surgeon of the Viconte de Rohan, who commanded a company of fifty cavalry. The counts Sancerre and de Jarnac each commanded similar detachments and these secured the wings of the camp.

On the route of the army the country people gathered in the towns and castles, taking their provisions with them. Living on the country, the huge cavalcade of the army found food very scarse; on three separate occasions, Ambroise thought he would die of hunger. Trying to buy food, a servant of one of M. de Rohan's officers went with a group of friends to a church where the peasants had retreated. When they were refused food, a fight ensued; the army servants were bested. The man of de Rohan's group was the most severely injured. He had seven sword wounds on his head, four on the arms and one that cut through half of the scapula. On his return, his master considered him moribund; a grave was dug for him and he was to have been thrown into it on the resumption of march, rather than left to be tortured and killed by the half-savage peasants. Pitying the servant in his desperate plight, Paré told the master that the man might be saved with proper dressing. Other Gentlemen urged the master to let the wounded man be taken along in the baggage, if Paré would agree to treat him. He

THE DEVELOPMENT OF THE MILITARY SURGEON 61

readily assented. A cart was prepared with a bed. Ambroise reported that he served the man in the capacities of physician, apothecary, surgeon and cook, and "God healed him." The men of the three companies were so impressed with the cure and the care that Paré gave the helpless servant, that at the first muster, each of de Rohan's men-at-arms gave him a crown, and each of the archers half a crown. (Malgaigne, III, p. 697; Hamby, p. 168).

On 13 April, 1552, the King was in Toul, and the next day was in Nancy, a distance of 24 km. On the 15th, Metz opened

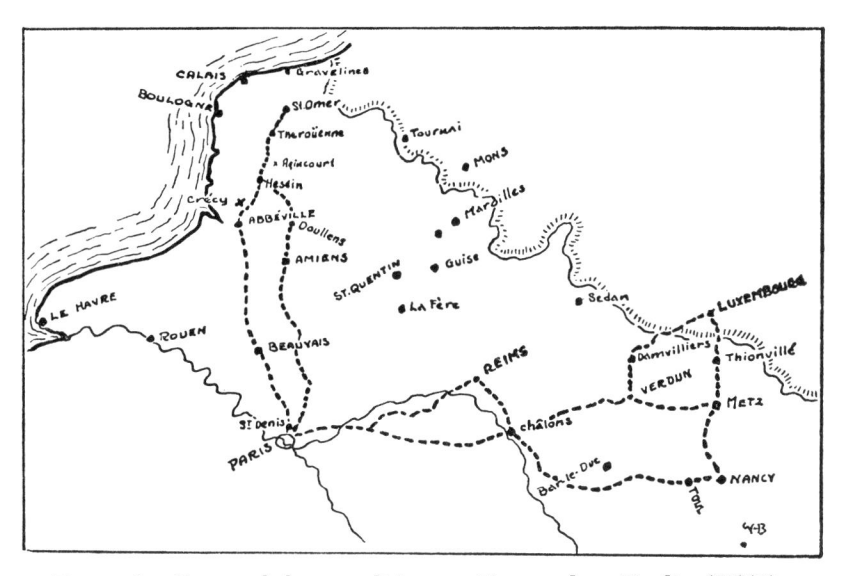

Figure 8. Route of the expeditions to Metz and to Hesdin (1552).

her gates, after a little hesitation. This was very rapid progress for so large a force. Henri thereafter retired to Verdun. While this had been more of a triumphal procession than a war, Henri had his troops in the field at the Emperors doorstep. By 1 June, the army set out for Luxembourg. On its return it encountered the fortified chateau town of Damvilliers. The inhabitants would not yield, so siege was laid down. Before the town could be taken, the French gunners ran out of powder and had to send back to Sedan for a fresh supply.

DAMVILLIERS

Paré described this campaign in his *Journeys* (Malgaigne, III, p. 698; Hamby, p. 169). Here he first used the ligature, instead of the customary cautery, to control hemorrhage during amputations. He had advised the cautery in his book on *Gunshot Wounds* published this same year, but had wondered about the propriety of using ligatures instead. He discussed the matter with de la Rivière and with François Rasse, of the College of Surgeons (Malgaigne, II, p. 230; Hamby, p. 73); they had agreed that it was worth trying. Here he had his first opportunity, but reserved reporting it until 1564, in his *Ten Books of Surgery*. By that time he had so proved its value that he advised complete abandonment of the cautery for this purpose.

A cannon ball from the enemy camp passed through M. de Rohan's tent, striking a Gentleman in the leg. It was necessary for Paré to finish removal of the member; he ligated the blood vessels instead of cauterizing them. The Gentlemen recovered and on breaking up of the camp on 26 July, Paré accompanied him to his house in Paris, "merry with a wooden leg, happy to have got off so cheap, and not miserably burned," as was usual in such cases. Unwittingly, Paré was leaving his friend de Rohan for the last time; on 4 November the Viconte was killed in the fighting at St. Nicholas, near Nancy.

Ambroise spent the summer in Paris, but great events were impending. The Emperor indicated a determination to retake Metz, so in August Henri put the thirty-three-year-old Duke de Guise into the city with troops and supplies to defend it. Guise prepared the city for her ordeal admirably. When the Duke d'Alva[53] reached the city on 19 October with twenty-four thousand Spaniards, Guise closed the gates—Metz was ready for her bid for glory. On 30 October, Alva began the assault; the Emperor was still twenty miles away at Thionville, ill with the gout.

CHÂTEAU-LE-COMTE

Paré's soujourn in Paris was not a prolonged one this time. To prevent the English from taking the opportunity to invade

Picardy, Henri raised an army of thirty thousand men to send into that area to lay it waste, making it difficult for a prospective invader to find subsistence there. As commander of this force he selected Antoine de Bourbon, then Duke de Vendôme, and made him King's Lieutenant. The Duke was at St. Denis, just north of Paris, while the companies passed northward, and he called Paré to him there. He asked Ambroise to go with him on this campaign, and as Paré said (Malgaigne, III, p. 699), his request was a command. His enthusiasm for army life probably having worn a little thin by this time, Paré tried to beg off; his wife was sick abed, etc. The Duke responded that there were physicians in Paris who could treat her, and that he also had left at home a wife probably as well born as Paré's own. He promised to use Ambroise well and to lodge him in his own train. In short, there was no way out of it and Ambroise promised to meet him at Château-le-Comte, three or four leagues from Hesdin, between Boulogne and Abbeville, about twenty kilometers from the Channel coast. Interestingly, this town lies about half-way between the old French-English battlefields of Crécy and Agincourt.

The French found Château-le-Comte occupied by Imperial troops, and the Duke de Vendôme called upon them to surrender. They refused, relying for protection upon a moat full of water. The Duke pounded a breach in the walls with his artillery and, after filling the moat with barrels and fagots, the infantry swarmed in. Seeing themselves taken, the defenders exploded their ammunition, burning many of their own men along with the attackers. The survivors were put to the sword, no quarter being. The French soldiers took twenty or thirty prisoners, hoping to get ransom for them. Learning of this, the Duke sent trumpets through the camp ordering that all Spanish prisoners taken were to be killed immediately, on pain of hanging and strangling. The order was executed at once, to Paré's dismay. Then the army beat the countryside, burning the villages and barns full of grain, to Paré great grief. They went as far as "Tournahan." This town I haven't been able to locate. It could be Tournai, now in Belgium, east of Lille. There was a great tower there that had been occupied earlier by the enemy, but it was found pillaged and deserted. The French mined the foundations and blew it over with gunpowder.

Their mission accomplished, the army was disbanded. Paré returned to Paris. There he found that his old friend, de Héry, had finally got his book on veneral diseases published. It was entitled *Méthode curatoire de la Maladie vénérienne*. From it, Paré was to borrow much of the material for his own remarks on the subject in his later books.

True to his promise, the Duke de Vendôme did very well by Ambroise. The day after the fall of Château-le-Comte the Duke sent a complete report of Paré's activities to the King, commending him highly on his surgical skill, remarking that Ambroise had shown him eighteen bullets he had removed from the wounded. Paré wrote that the Duke said more good of him than was actually necessary. As a result, the King decided that he wanted Ambroise in his service. He ordered his Premier-Physician, Dr. de Gaugier, to record Paré as a Surgeon-in-Ordinary and to order him to Reims within ten or twelve days to take up his commission by the King. Henri ordered him to remain near him and promised to see that he was well taken care of. Ambroise thanked him humbly for the honor bestowed upon him by calling him into his service.

This was indeed a signal honor. Although Henri had a number of barber-surgeons in his service, they were a highly selected group. This rank gave them equality with the educated surgeons in the corps and indicated that the included barber-surgeons were men of exceptional ability.

The new post brought additional responsibilities, as well as increased opportunities. As a member of the King's household, Ambroise was now privileged and required to spend a certain portion of his time near the King's person, not only on military campaigns but also in his residence with the Court. He was in intimate contact with the most powerful of the military chiefs and politicians, the most educated and cultured of the writers, philosophers and poets, the western world's cleverest diplomats, the leaders of the Church, and the most brilliant, beautiful and ambitious women in France. In addition to the finest and the best in the country, he was also exposed to the most successful of the clever, unscrupulous and ambitious knaves in the kingdom. Only his own character determined the influences by which a man so placed would be molded.

While the royal service had first call upon his time and energies, the new post was not a full time job. Between his assignments, Paré had the opportunity to live in his own house in his periods off duty, to continue his private practice and to carry on his own schedule of investigation and writing.

CHAPTER V

King's Surgeon; The Great Sieges
1552-1553

METZ

THE EMPEROR finally arrived at Metz with sixty thousand men on 20 November, 1552. Although still pale and weak from his last bout with the gout, he put on a good show and arrived on a splended white Arabian charger.

The winter of 1552 was an unusually severe one; it became formidable in November and worse in December. Metz is situated on the triangle in the confluence of the Moselle and Sielle rivers, forcing the besiegers to deploy between these channels to attack on the open face of the fork. The Imperial troops were encamped in a swamp and, as Paré wrote in his splendid account (Malgaigne, III, p. 708), they were beaten by the cold, hunger and the plague. He said the snow was two feet deep and the soldiers lived in caves in the ground, covered only by a little straw.

> Nevertheless, each soldier had his field bed with a covering strewn with glittering stars, brighter than fine gold. Every day they had white sheets and lodged at the Sign of the Moon. They made good cheer when they had it, and paid their host so well over night that in the morning they went away quit, shaking their ears. They needed no comb to get the down out of the hair of either head or beard. They always found a white tablecloth, missing good meals only for want of victuals. Also most of them had neither boots nor buskins, slippers, hose nor shoes. Many preferred not to have them, since they always were in the mud halfway up the leg, and because they went bare-legged, we called them "The Emperor's Apostles."

KING'S SURGEON; THE GREAT SIEGES 67

One of the most intimate accounts of the siege and Paré's part in it was his own, written in his *Journeys* (Malgaigne, III, pp. 700-708). Perhaps, it would be best to let him tell it here:

The Emperor besieged Metz in the depth of winter, as everyone remembers. In the city were five or six thousand men, including seven Princes, M. le duc de Guise the King's Lieutenant, Messieurs d'Anguien,[54] de Conde,[55] de Montpensier,[56] de la Roche-sur-Yon,[57] de Nemours,[58] and many other Gentlemen and Captains-at-War. They often made sallies upon the enemy (as we shall describe later), which resulted in many deaths on each side. Most of our wounded died, and it was believed that the medicaments used in dressing were poisoned. For that reason, the duc de Guise and other Princes sent to the King for me to bring them fresh drugs. I don't believe there was any poison, the reason was the great cutlass wounds, musket shot, and the severe cold. The King wrote the Mareschal St. Andre, his Lieutenant at Verdun, that means be found to get me into Metz. Msrs. le Mareschal St. Andre and le Mareschal de Villeville[59] found an Italian Captain who promised to get me in, which he did, for which he got 1500 crowns. Learning of the Italian Captain's promise, the King sent for me and ordered me to get from his Apothecary, named Daigue, such and as many drugs as I thought necessary for the wounded besieged, which I did, as much as a post horse could carry. The King gave me messages to carry to M. de Guise and to the Princes and Captains who were in Metz.

Arriving in Verdun a few days later, M. de St. Andre got horses for me, for my man and for the Italian Captain, who spoke very good German, Spanish and Walloon, as well as his own tongue. When we got within 8 or 10 leagues of Metz, we traveled only by night and when approaching the camp I saw a league and a half of fires burning around the city, appearing as if the earth were on fire. I thought we would never pass through those fires without being discovered and consequently hanged, strangled, cut to pieces, or obliged to pay a big ransom. Truly, I fondly wished myself back in Paris, for the great danger I foresaw. God guided our affairs so well that we entered the city at midnight by means of a certain signal between the Captain and another Captain of the company of M. de Guise. I went to this Lord, whom I found in bed, but he received me with good grace, being very happy over my arrival. I delivered to him the message containing all the King had ordered me to tell him. I told him I had a little letter to give him and that I would not fail to deliver it the next day. He then ordered that I be given good lodging and that I should be well used. He told me that I should not fail the next day to be on the breach where I would find all the Princes and Lords and many Captains, which I did. They received me with great joy and did me the honor of embracing me and saying that I was welcome, adding that they no longer feared dying, should they happen to be wounded.

    M. de la Roche-sur-Yon was the first to feast me and inquired what was said at the Court of the city of Metz; I told him what I thought proper. Then he asked me to go see one of his Gentlemen, M. de Magnane, now Chevalier of the Order of the King and Lieutenant of His Majesty's Guard, whose leg had been broken by a cannon shot. I found him in his bed, his leg bent and crooked, with no dressing on it, because a certain Gentleman had promised to cure him with certain words, taking his name and girdle. The poor Gentleman wept and cried with pain, sleeping neither night nor day for four days. I mocked at this false imposture. I quickly set and dressed his leg so dextrously that he was free of pain and slept through the night. Thanks to God, he was cured and still lives, serving the King. The said Prince de la Roche-sur-Yon sent a tun of wine, larger than a pipe of Anjou, to my lodgings and had me told that when it was drunk, he would send me another. That was how he treated me, making me all good cheer.

  That done, M. de Guise gave me a list of certain Captains and Lords and ordered me to tell them what the King had given me in charge, which I did. This was, to commend them and to thank them for the duty they had done and were doing in defending his city of Metz, and that he would remember it. I was more than eight days in discharging my duty, they were so many. First of all, to the Princes and others, such as the duc Horace,[60] the Comte de Martigues[61] and his brother M. de Bauge, the Lords Montmorency and d'Anville, now Mareschal of France, M. de la Chapelle des Ursins, Bonnivet, Carouge, now Governor of Rouen, the Vidame de Chartres,[62] the Comte de Lude, M. de Biron, now Mareschal of France, M. de Randan, la Rochefoucauld, Bordaille, d'Estres the younger, M. de St.

Jean-en-Dauphine, and others too many to mention, even to the Captains who all had done their duty well in defense of their lives and of the town. Later I asked M. de Guise what I should do with the drugs I had brought. He told me to divide them among the surgeons and the apothecaries and especially to the many poor wounded soldiers at the Hotel-Dieu, which I did. I can assure you that I could not visit all the wounded who sent for me to come see and dress them.

All the besieged Lords besought me to care most solicitously above all for M. de Pienne, who had been wounded on the breach by a fragment of stone shot from a cannon, in the temple with a fracture and depression of the bone. They told me that immediately upon being struck, he fell to the ground as if dead, bleeding from his mouth, nose and ears and vomiting profusely. For fourteen days, he was unable to speak or reason and he developed tremors like spasms, his face swollen and livid. He was trepanned at the side of the temporal muscle on the frontal bone (by Pierre Aubert,[64] then surgeon of the Duke de Guise, later King's Surgeon-in-Ordinary; see Malgaigne II, p. 63). I dressed him with other surgeons and God cured him. He is still living today, thank God.

The Emperor had a battery of 40 double cannon set up, where powder was not spared by day or night. As soon as M. de Guise saw the artillery set and pointed to make a breach, he had the nearest houses pulled down to make ramparts. The posts and beams were put end-to-end and between them faggots, earth, beds and bales of rags, then other beams and joints were set over them. Now, much of the wood of the suburban houses that had been pulled down (for fear the enemy would lodge in cover there and use the wood) served very well to repair the breach. Everybody was busy day and night carrying earth to repair the breach. Messieurs the Princes, Lords, Captains, Leiutenants and Ensigns, all were carrying baskets to give example to the soldiers and civilians to do the same, which they did, even ladies and gentlewomen. Those who had no baskets used caldrons, panniers, sacks, sheets and anything they could find to carry earth, so the enemy had no sooner beaten down the wall that he found a stronger rampart behind it. The wall having fallen, our soldiers cried 'fox, fox, fox' to those outside and called a thousand insults upon them. M. de Guise forbade, under pain of death, any man talking to those outside, for fear of traitors informing them what was being done. At his prohibition, they tied live cats to their pikes and putting them on the wall, cried 'Meiou, meiou, meiou' with the cats. Truly, the Imperials were enraged, having been so long and at such great expense at making a breach, which was eighty paces wide, that fifty men could enter abreast, when they saw a rampart stronger than the wall. They threw themselves upon the poor cats and shot at them with arquebuses as one shoots at popinjays.

Our people often made sorties at the order of M. de Guise. The day before, there was a great rush to enroll among those to go out, especially among the young noblemen, led by veteran Captains, so it was a great privilege to be permitted to sally out and run against the enemy. They would sally out a hundred to six score, well armed with bucklers, cutlasses, arbuebuses and pistols, pikes, partisans and halberds, going as far as the trenches to awaken them in surprise. There the alarm would go through the camp and their drums would sound, 'plan, plan, ta ti ta, ta ta ti ta, tou, touf, touf!' Likewise their trumpets and clarions roared and sang, 'To saddle, to saddle, to saddle— to horse, to horse, to saddle, to horse' and the soldiers would cry, 'Arm, arm, arm, to arms, to arms, to arms, arm, to arms, arm, to arms, arm, to arms, arms,' as one cries after wolves, and all in different languages, according to their nations. One saw them rush out of their tents and little huts as thick as ants when one uncovers their anthills, to help their companions who were having their throats cut like sheep. The cavalry likewise came from all sides at a great gallop, 'Patati, patati, patati, patata, pa, ta, ta, patata, pata, ta,' eager to be in the melee where the strokes were falling, to give and to receive them. And when ours saw themselves pressed, they returned to the town, fighting constantly and their pursuers were repulsed by the artillery, charged with stones and great square and three sided pieces of iron. Our soldiers on the wall would fire a volley and rain bullets upon them, thick as hail, to send them back to bed. But many remained upon the fields of combat and our men did not always return with whole skins. Some always remained behind for the tax, glad to die on the field of honor. If a horse was wounded, it was skinned by the soldiers and eaten instead of beef or bacon, and it was up to me to run and dress our wounded. Sometimes, sorties were made on the next day, which greatly vexed the enemy that we would not let them sleep a little safely.

M. de Guise made a strategem, or a ruse of war. He sent a peasant, who was not very bright, with two letters to the King. He gave him ten ecus and promised that the King would give him a hundred if he delivered the letter to him. In one of the letters, he said that the enemy gave no sign of retiring and that his forces had made a great breach, which he hoped to defend even to the loss of his own life and that of those with him. And, that if the enemy had put his artillery in a certain place he designated, only with great difficulty could he keep him from entering, since it was the weakest place in the whole city, but that he hoped soon to repair it so they could not enter. This letter was sewed into the lining of the peasant's doublet and he was told that he must say nothing of it to anyone. He was given another in which M. de Guise told the King that he and all the besieged hoped to defend the town well and other things I will leave unsaid here. He sent the peasant out into the night and he was taken by a sentinel and was brought to the duc d'Alva to learn what was done in the town. They asked him if he had letters: he said 'yes' and gave them one. Having seen it, they asked on oath if he had others and he said he had not. Then they searched him and found the one sewed into his doublet, and the poor messenger was hanged and strangled.

The said letters were communicated to the Emperor, who called the Council, where it was resolved that since they had not been able to do anything at the first breach, the artillery should be brought quickly to the place they thought the weakest. There they made great efforts to make another breach; they sapped and mined the walls and sought to surprise the Hell Tower, yet they dared not come to the assault.

The duc d'Alva reproached the Emperor that his soldiers were dying, as many as two hundred a day and that, thanks to the weather and the number of soldiers in the town, there was little hope of entering it. The Emperor demanded what men were dying, and if they Gentlemen and men of mark. He was answered that they were all poor soldiers. He said then that it did not matter if they did die, comparing them to caterpillars, grasshoppers and cockchafers which eat the buds and other good things of earth, saying that if they were men of worth they would not be in his camp at six livres a month; therefore no harm was done if they did die. Moreover, he said, he would not leave the town before he had taken it by force or famine, even if he should lose his entire army, because of the great number of Princes confined there, with the greatest part of the French nobility, whom he hoped would pay his expenses quadrupled. He would go yet once more to Paris to visit the Parisians and to make himself King of the entire French kingdom.

M. de Guise, with the Princes, Captains and soldiers and, in general, all the citizens of the town, hearing the intentions of the Emperor to exterminate all of us, prohibited the soldiers and civilians and even the Princes and Lords to eat fresh fish or venison, partridges, woodcocks, larks, plovers, divers and other game, for fear they might have acquired some pestilence which might give us a contagion. They must be content with army fare; to wit, biscuit, beef, salted cow, bacon, sausage, Mayence hams, such fish as mollusks, haddock, salmon, shad, tunny, whale, anchovy, sardines, herring, and peas, beans, rice, garlic, onions, prunes, cheeses, butter, oil and salt, pepper, ginger, nutmeg and other spices to put into our pastries, chiefly of horsemeat, without which they had a very bad flavor. Many citizens with gardens in the town had planted them with fine radishes, turnip, carrots and leeks, which they guarded well and dearly against the extreme necessity of hunger. But all these supplies were distributed justly by weight and measure according to the quality of the persons, because we did not know how long the siege would last. Because it had been heard from the mouth of the Emperor that he would never leave Metz until he had taken it by force, the victuals were retrenched, so that what had been given to three soldiers was given to four. They were forbidden to sell what remained of their meals, but were permitted to give it to the camp-followers. They always arose from the table with an appetite, for fear they would be subjected to taking medicine. Before giving ourselves up to the enemy, we determined to eat the asses, mules and horses, dogs, cats and rats, and even our boots, collars and other leathers we could stew and soften.

In general, all the besieged were determined to defend themselves valorously with all the instruments of war; to point and charge the artillery at the site of the breach with bullets, stones, cart nails, iron bars, and chains; also all types and kinds of firearms, such as boëttes, barricades, grenades, pots, lances, torches and fuses, circles surrounded by caltrops, burning faggots, boiling water, melted lead and quick-lime to put out their eyes. Also, they made openings from one side to the other through the houses to lodge arquebusiers to fight them on the flanks and to hasten their going, or make them stay there forever. Moreover, the women were commissioned to pull up the paving blocks and to haul these 'St. Stephen's loaves,' billets, tables, trestles, benches and stools which would dash out their brains.

In addition, near the front there was a great guard house filled with carts and pallisades, casks and barrels and barricades filled with earth to serve as gabions, interlaid with falconets and falcons, field pieces, arquebuses with barrel-rests, arquebuses and pistols and artifices of fire which would break legs and thighs, so they would be attacked at the head, in the flanks and in the rear. Had they forced this guard house, there were more yet at the street crossings at every hundred paces, which would have been as bad as the first or worse. They would have made many widows and orphans and if fortune had been so much against us, that they had stormed and broken our guardhouses, there would yet have been seven great battalions drawn up in square and triangle to fight all together, each accompanied by a Prince to embolden them to fight all together, to the last breath of their souls. In addition, they all resolved that each would carry his treasure, rings and jewels, his best, richest and most beautiful furniture, and burn them to ashes in the great square to prevent the enemy from getting them as trophies, should they prevail. Men were charged to set fire to and burn all the munitions and break in the wine vessels in the cellars. Others were detailed to set fire to every house to burn our enemies and ourselves together. The citizens ratified all this, rather than see the bloody knife at their throats and their wives and daughters taken by force and ravished by the cruel and inhuman Spaniards.

We had certain prisoners who were quietly permitted to understand our desperation and final resolution. M. de Guise released them on parole and on arriving in their camp, they lost no time in announcing it. This restrained the impetuosity of the soldiers to enter the town and cut our throats, since they would not enrich themselves by our pillage. Having heard the will of this great warrior, M. de Guise, the Emperor put water into his wine and restrained his rage. He said he could not enter the town without great butchery and carnage, shedding much blood, both of the defenders and their assailants who would all die together. In the end, he would have got nothing but ashes, and afterward men would compare this to the destruction of the city of Jerusalem, made earlier by Titus and Vespasian.

Having thus heard our last resolution and seeing how little he had gained by his battery, saps and mines, the great plague throughout his camp, the inclement weather, the lack of food and money, and how the soldiers were deserting in great troops, the Emperor decided at last to retire, accompanied by the cavalry of his advance guard, with the greater part of the artillery and the engines of war. The Marquis of Brandenberg was the last to decamp, sustained by some bands of Spaniards, Bohemians and his Germans. He remained for a day and a half, to the annoyance of M. de Guise, who sent four pieces of artillery out of the town to fire upon them at random to hasten his going, which he did soon enough, with all his troops. When a quarter of a league from Metz, he took flight, fearing our cavalry would fall upon his rear. This caused him to set fire to his munition powder and abandon some pieces of artillery and much baggage, which he could not transport, since the roads had been cut to pieces by the advance guard, the machines of war and the great cannon. Our cavalry wanted with all their might to go out and attack his rear, but M. de Guise would not permit it. On the contrary, he said, we should rather smooth the roads for them and make gold and silver bridges for them, like a good pastor and shepherd who did not wish to lose a single one of his flock.

That is how our dear and well-beloved Imperialists went away from Metz the day before Christmas, to the joy of the Princes and Seigneurs, Captains and soldiers who had endured the travail of this siege for two months. Yet, they did not all go; there lacked more than twenty-thousand who had died by artillery and the sword, as well as by the plague and the cold and hunger (and from spite and rage that they could not get into the city to pillage it and cut our throats). Also, a great number of their horses had died, most of which they ate instead of beef or bacon. We went where they had camped, where we found many dead bodies not yet buried, with the earth all dug up as we see in the Cemetery of the Holy Innocents during some great mortality. In their tents, pavilions and lodgings, they also had left many sick; also bullets, arms, carts, wagons and other baggage, with a great quantity of munition bread spoiled and rotted by the snows, yet the soldiers got it only by weight and measure. They also left a great store of wood, the remains of the houses they had demolished and torn down in the villages for two and three leagues around, as well as many villas belonging to citizens with gardens and fine orchards filled with various fruit trees. Without this they all would have been dead and numb with the cold and forced to raise the siege earlier.

M. de Guise had the dead buried and the sick treated. The enemy had left in the Abbey of St. Arnold many of their wounded soldiers whom they had no means of taking away. M. de Guise sent them plenty of food and ordered me and the other surgeons to dress and treat them, which we did with a good will. I believe they would not have done the same for ours, for the Spaniard is very cruel, perfidious and inhuman, and therefore the enemy of all nations. This is proved by Lopez the Spaniard and Benzo the Milanese, and others who have written the history of America and the West Indes. They have had to confess that the cruelty, avarice, blasphemy and wickedness of the Spaniards have altogether alienated the poor Indians from the religion the said Spaniards are said to profess. All write that they are less worthy than the idolatrous Indians, for their cruel treatment of the said Indians.

After some days we sent a trumpet to Thionville to the enemy, that they should send in safety for their wounded, which they did, with too few carts and wagons. M. de Guise gave them carts and carters to help take them to Thionville. On their return, our carters told us that the roads were paved with dead bodies and half never arrived, since they had died in the carts. Seeing them at the point of death, the Spaniards cast them out of the carts and buried them in the mud and mire before they had drawn their last breaths, saying that they had no orders to bring back the dead. The carters also reported finding by the road many carts laden with baggage stuck in the mud, which the enemy dared not send for, fearing that those in Metz would run against them.

After the camp was entirely broken up, I distributed my sick in the hands of surgeons in the town to continue their care. I took leave of M. de Guise and returned to the King, who received me with a good countenance and asked me how I had got into the city of Metz. I told him entirely all I had done. He gave me 200 ecus and the 100 I had at setting, and said that he would never leave me poor. Then I thanked him humbly for the good and honor he was pleased to do me.

Naturally, many accounts have been written of this epic fight and Paré figures in several of them in greater or lesser detail and in some with very debatable accuracy. When Malgaigne wrote in 1840, he was considerably impressed by word-of-mouth reports on data said to be in the hands of Dr. Emilé Bégin of Metz. In 1878-1879, Dr. Bégin published a series of four articles allegedly based upon a small, 122 page journal he saw in Metz, said to have been written in Paré's own hand. Le Paulmier denied the authenticity of the journal; its style and language were not in keeping with those of Ambroise, and statements could be disproved from other sources. In this journal, Paré was described as leaving Metz on a fine bay horse given him by M. de Guise, with his man, in a company of French officers. Taking three days to get to Verdun, they were entertained there by the Franciscan fathers, since the town was overrun by refugees. They inspected hospitals, performed a number of operations and finally took the old road leading straight to Reims. Back in Paris, about the end of January 1553, Paré resumed his work in anatomy. Thierry de Héry no longer was with him; he had as assistant a sworn-surgeon of Paris, Rostan or Rostaing de Binosc[65] from Provence, who stayed with him for several years.

In the spring of 1553, the Emperor moved westward through Picardy, smarting from his insult at Metz and itching for a chance to even accounts with Henri. Believing he had completely ruined his and his late father's arch-enemy, Henri paid little attention to his activities. The country shared the King's disdain and inattention. The Court was in a mood of merrymaking, concentrating on the grand festivities attending the wedding of

Henri's illegitimate Piedmontese daughter, Diane de France, to the Duke Horace Farnese, one of the heros of Metz. In addition, Catherine de' Médicis had had another baby at St. Germain-en-Laye on 14 May. This was Marguerite, later to become the famous Queen Margot, who would marry Henri de Bourbon, future King Henri IV.

Suddenly, news reached Paris that the Emperor's army was laying siege to Therouenne, an important fortress between Artois and Picardy, guarding the road to Calais. The Duke de Savoy[66] had invested the place which, despite its importance, was defended only lightly by a small force. On 19 June, d'Alva mounted a sanguinary assault and, on the advice of his officers, François de Montmorency, the Constable's son who was in command, offered surrender. Unfortunately, the inexperienced young man failed to bargain for terms and opened the castle unconditionally. Fresh from their defeat at Metz, the Germans and Spaniards pillaged the place, captured the officers and slaughtered the soldiers. François de Montmorency himself remained the Emperor's prisoner for three years until released under the terms of the Treaty of Vaucelles, signed on 5 February, 1556. On the order of the Emperor, the fortress was systematically demolished until, as Paré wrote later, a cart could be driven over the area without finding a remnant of the fort. The Emperor was in Brussels when he heard the news and the Netherlands rang with the celebration of this morsel of revenge after his recent defeat. Looking for another quick victory to bolster the sagging morale of his Empire, he sent Savoy against the neighboring château-fort of Hesdin, 45 kilometers south of Therouenne.

HESDIN

Anticipating this move and by now thoroughly alarmed at the fall of Therouenne, Henri sent eighteen hundred soldiers under the Duke of Bouillon, the bridegroom Horace, M. de Martiques and the Marquis de Villars to strengthen the château of Hesdin. Paré went with them. They worked so earnestly that by the first of July the place seemed impregnable and the defenders settled down for the siege. Savoy struck hard almost immediately. Paré described this siege in detail almost as meticulous (Malgaigne, III, pp. 709-720) as that used in the case of Metz.

Hesdin now is a sleepy little Flemish town of thirty-five hundred people on the bank of the river Canche, with only its big paved "grand-place" marking the site of the earlier huge château. In the Hôtel-de-France is a small octagonal room supposed to have been Paré's operating room, but his own description of the siege proves this erroneous; not that much of the château was left standing and it is much too near the river. Hesdin is surrounded by the wheat fields of Picardy, cut into wooded ravines by meandering streams. Paré told of standing on a rampart by a cannon watching a hundred or so enemy camp-followers and wenches beside one of these streams. Having acquired a military curiosity by now, he asked M. du Pont, the Artillery Chief, if he could reach the camp with his gun. The answer was a contemptuous affirmative, but with the remark that these people were not worth the required cannon powder. Ambroise replied that they could be quick with the knife when the time came, and "the more dead, the fewer enemies." At that the gun fired, killing fifteen or sixteen of them and wounding many others.

As at Metz, the defenders ran raiding sorties against the enemy camp frequently, so Paré was busy day and night dressing the wounded. He described how the wounded were hospitalized in a great tower with only a little straw to protect them from the stone floors. When the big guns were fired, the concussion was transmitted to their bodies, tormenting their painful wounds and causing some to bleed afresh, requiring redressing to control the hemorrhage. The defenders did not have the reserve food stocks they had enjoyed at Metz and subsisted on poor fare, poorly salted beef, etc., that was difficult for even the healthy to eat. In his account addressed to his Faculty adversary, Gourmelen, he "supposed" ironically that had he been there, he would have ordered fine diets for his patients to speed their recoveries, but the food was not available. And, had he used the cautery he so strongly advised in his book to control hemorrhage, "they would have killed you like a calf for your cruelty."

He described the rags they were forced to use for dressings, rewashed daily and dried over a fire until they were as stiff as parchment. Four "big, fat prostitutes" were detailed to the task of washing, but they had no soap and little water, so they could do little more than beat them with sticks in muddy water. They could not get to the nearby river and had only one well, which was nearly dried up. The water became so thick they had to strain it before it could be drunk.

Once the enemy made an attack on the breach to draw out the defenders for reconnoitering them. A priest of the Duke de Bouillon, attempting to throw a grenade at the enemy, let it explode in a supply of their fire artifices. Beyond the effect of burning a number of French soldiers, it almost produced a major calamity, since it set fire to the house, in the face of the water shortage. They extinguished it with beer, however, averting a more serious holocaust. Seeing this brave display of fireworks, the attackers abandoned the attack on the breach, thinking the French must have plenty more fire in reserve. They sapped and mined the walls then, causing the château to shake as if in an earthquake when the guns were fired.

Paré was called to see a Gentleman of M. d'Estampes company (Malgaigne, II, p. 22; Hamby, p. 25) who had been on the breach and was knocked down by an arquebus shot that struck his helmet. The helmet was dented, but there was no scalp wound. The man was unconscious and on the sixth day, died in convulsions. Curious of the mechanism of such an injury, Paré did an autopsy and found the brain lacerated by bone fragments driven in from the inner table of the skull, while the outer was not fractured.

On another occasion (Malgaigne, II, p. 39; Hamby, p. 32), he saw a soldier who had been digging from a pit earth to take to the ramparts. The walls of the pit caved in upon him and his companions pulled him out. His scalp was cut down to the pericranium, the wound starting two inches below the vertex of the head; the scalp flap hanging over his face gave him a horrible appearance. Ambroise called Charles Lambert, the Duke of Bouillon's surgeon, to help him. They washed out the dirt with warm wine and stitched the scalp back with several loose sutures. The head was dressed to favor drainage. The man did well and before the final assault was made on the castle, he was transferred to Abbeville where he could get better treatment.

The Duke Horace, that ill-fated bridegroom, was struck by a cannon ball in the shoulder (see Malgaigne, III, p. 710; Hamby, p. 170), lopping off the arm and killing him instantly. This had a disastrous effect on the morale of the place, since the Duke was a man of high rank and authority. Then, M. de Martigues leaned over a wall to watch the enemy sapping the foundations (Malgaigne, III, p. 710; Hamby, p. 171). He was shot through the chest by an arquebus ball and Paré was called to see him. He was coughing up blood and the chest wound bled freely. He had trouble breathing, the motion causing air to whistle in and out of the wounds of entrance and exit. The wound, at the level of the fourth and fifth ribs, hurt severely and Paré found the ribs smashed into fragments, some of which he removed. He plugged the wounds with large linen tents annointed with a mixture of egg yolks, Venice turpentine and oil of roses, essentially the same mixture he had used as his emergency dressing for the gunshot wounds at Turin. He fastened cords to them so they could be withdrawn should they happen to be pulled into the chest by respiratory movements. He then covered the chest with a big plaster, bandaged to somewhat splint the chest. The Count continued to expectorate blood, from which Paré deduced that the lung was injured by the ball and by the rib fragments. He knew this was liable to get worse, because of the constant motion of the lung. The Count also evacuated a large amount of blood by bladder and bowel (Malgaigne II, p. 195; Hamby, p. 68), promptly developed a fever and his heart grew weak, so Paré realized he was doomed to die within a few days.

The surviving commanders then sent a herald to the Duke de Savoy, asking terms for surrender. They were told that the Gentlemen, Captains, Lieutenants and Ensigns would be held for ransom, while the soldiers could go free unarmed. They added that this was their best offer, for tomorrow they would storm and take the place. A Council of War was held, to which

Ambroise was asked, to vote on acceptance of the terms. Paré told them that he would sign the surrender in his own blood if necessary, since he considered the place untenable. He was at the end of his endurance, having slept neither night nor day for a long period, due to the pressure of caring for almost two hundred wounded. When he went through a door he could not put foot to ground, but was carried "like a holy body" from one wounded man to the next. He protested that he could not do his duty to them because of their numbers and supplies inadequate to dress them. The dead were another source of great menace. No burial space was available and bodies were stacked like firewood in a tower, putrefying in the July heat.

After the decision was made to surrender, Paré decided to disguise himself in order to avoid having to pay a heavy ransom. He traded his velvet coat, satin doublet and velvet-lined cloak with a poor soldier in exchange for his own worn doublet, a tattered leather collar, a short coat and a miserable hat. He rubbed soot into his skin and, with a stone, abraded his shoes and his hose at the knees and heels to simulate long wear. As he said, he more nearly resembled a chimney-sweep than a King's surgeon. He went in this disguise to M. de Martigues and asked if he could go with him to dress him. The Count was as happy to have him as Ambroise was to go.

On July 17, the Imperial Commission charged with choosing the prisoners entered the château. They took with them Messrs. the Duke de Bouillon, the Marquis de Villars, de Roye, the Baron de Culan, M. du Pont and M. de Martigues with Paré, Gentlemen they knew could pay ransom, and a number of lesser military officers. Then the Spanish soldiers came pouring in to plunder and to kill, regardless of terms of surrender. Paré described some of the fiendish tortures inflicted upon those suspected of trying to evade ransom. If the tormenters were not satisfied with the victim's answers, they cut his throat on the spot. In the end they were all murdered, another cipher added to the mental score Paré kept of the savagery of the Spaniards.

Ambroise was taken with M. de Martiques into the town where a Gentleman asked him if his employer would recover from his wound. Paré told him that the Count was mortally wounded. The Gentleman hurried to M. de Savoy with the news, since a good ransom was being expected from the patient. Paré was in a quandary then, whether to play the simpleton at the risk of being murdered, or to reveal himself as a surgeon. The latter course might result in his being impressed into duty to help with the enemy wounded, and he might be forced to pay a large ransom for his freedom. He decided then to show that the Count would not die because of improper attention, and to let events care for the future.

Soon they were visited by many Gentlemen, a physician and a surgeon of the Emperor, as well as those of the Duke de Savoy, and six other army surgeons. They wanted to see the Count's wounds and to find out how he had been dressed. The Emperor's physician ordered Paré to declare the essential nature of the wound and how it had been managed. The others listened carefully, to make their own prognoses. Ambroise gave them a real lecture on the physiology of thoracic wounds and his conception of the pathology in this particular case. He then dressed the wounds in their presence and they agreed with his conclusions.

They returned to the Duke de Savoy then, with the sad news that the rumor was true; M. de Martigues was indeed mortally wounded and could survive but a short time. The Duke suggested that had he been better tended, he might have survived, but the professional people unanimously applauded the care Paré had given him, saying that no one could have done better. The Duke actually wept in his frustration.

Then a Spanish imposter came forward and told the Duke that he could cure the Count, if he were allowed to proceed in his own way without interference by the medical people and surgeons (Hamby, p. 175). He staked his life on it, saying that they could cut him into a thousand pieces if he failed. This was the best offer Savoy had heard, so he agreed and ordered the medical people to let the Spaniard alone. He sent a Gentleman to Paré, telling him not to touch the patient again at the price of his life. Secretly happy to be relieved of the responsibility and knowing that the Count had nothing to lose, Ambroise agreed. The Spaniard then came, telling the Count that he had been ordered to treat him. He swore by God that in eight days he would have him back on horseback, lance in hand, if he would follow his orders. He could eat and drink what he wanted; the Spaniard would diet for him. He told him that he had cured many worse hurt than he was. The poor Count rather wearily wished him God-speed.

The Spaniard took one of M. de Martigues' shirts and tore it into strips, which he arranged over the wounded area in the form of a cross, muttering incantations all the while. He then let the Count have all he wanted to eat and drink; he himself ate only a few prunes and six morsels of bread and drank a little beer. Nevertheless, two days later the Count died and the imposter fled. Paré believed that he would have been hanged for his stupid hoax, had he been found.

The Count died at ten o'clock in the morning and soon afterward came a procession of Gentlemen, physicians and surgeons to witness the autopsy and embalmment (Hamby, p. 172). The Emperor's surgeon asked Paré to do the work. It is likely that he had no proper idea of how to do it himself; the Spanish court did not approve of taking liberties with corpses. Ambroise demurred, saying that he was not worthy to carry the surgeon's instruments and that he should proceed. The surgeon then asked him to do it for friendship's sake. Paré again declined, asking that one of the other Spaniards do the autopsy if the surgeon did not wish to. The surgeon then ordered him to proceed, threatening him with unpleasant consequences if he refused. Finally, Paré saw that they were determined to watch him work, so he decided to give them a real lesson.

He started by telling them what he believed would be found, based on the symptoms and signs developed during life. Then, he opened the body and demonstrated everything exactly as anticipated, the broken ribs with the splinters directed by the passage of the ball, the blood in the thorax, the wide laceration in the collapsed lung, etc. He answered a number of questions posed by his audience, then embalmed the body and put it into a coffin.

After this demonstration, the Emperor's surgeon took Paré aside and attempted to enlist him in his service, promising him good treatment and a rich practice. Paré thanked him, but told him that he could not enter the service of a foreign Lord. The annoyed and disappointed surgeon called him a fool, saying that under the circumstances he would serve the devil himself to regain his freedom. The Emperor's physician (this was not Vesalius, who was in Brussels at the time, according to Cushing), went back to the Duke, reported the events of the autopsy, and urged him to take Paré into his service. The Duke sent M. de Bouchet, one of his Maitres-d'hôtel, to Paré and offered to take him into his service, promising him good treatment. Paré thanked him humbly for his offer, but again declined to enter foreign service. This angered the Duke, who said that he should send him to the galleys.

M. de Vaudeville, Governor of Gravelines, a town between Calais and Dunkerque, then asked the Duke to give Ambroise to him to treat a leg ulcer he had carried for several years (Malgaigne, III, p. 716; Hamby, p. 177). The Duke said he could have him and it would serve him right if Paré set his leg afire. The Governor promised to have his throat cut if he tried it. In a short time, four German halberdiers came to fetch Ambroise, who was quite perturbed, since he spoke no more German than they did French, and he had no idea where they were taking him. They took him to M. de Vaudeville, however, who welcome him and told him that he now belonged to him. He told Ambroise that he would release him without ransom if he would cure his leg ulcer. Paré replied that he had no means of paying ransom, but that he would cure the ulcer if he could.

Paré inspected the ulcer, with the Governor's physician and surgeon, then he retired with them and carefully outlined his plan of therapy for this indolent varicose ulcer. They found it to be an acceptable one, and so reported to the Governor. Ambroise then was called in and he and the Governor bargained over details. Ambroise was promised his freedom if he would cure the ulcer, and he could have this as soon as it was apparent that the cure was well on its way, not being required to remain until it was complete; this, the Governor swore on his word as a Gentleman. Paré outlined his projected treatment, which included a rigid diet, avoiding meat, wine and salted foods. It also required a change of activity and habits, rest and avoidance of emotional excess; to this the Governor agreed. Ambroise then cut two paper patterns of the dimensions of the ulcer, giving one to the Governor and keeping one for himself, to have objective evidence of the original status of the lesion.

Ambroise then started his therapy and dressed the ulcer daily. The patient and his inexperienced physician became impatient and in the patient's presence, the Doctor urged Paré to dress it more often. Ambroise asked that he be left alone; he had no desire to prolong the treatment; he was anxious to regain his freedom as rapidly as possible. He suggested that the physician read Galen's advise on the matter, quoting book and paragraph, that a frequently dressed wound heals slower than one less often disturbed. The Lord was curious about this quotation, coming from an apparently ignorant barber-surgeon, and sent the physician to get the book, to verify it. Paré's statement was found to be accurate, which made him happy, but embarrassed the physician. He had no more interference thereafter and within fifteen days the healing was well advanced.

Paré became more relaxed then and began enjoying himself. The Governor had him eat at his own table when no one of greater rank was present. He gave Ambroise more freedom, but made him wear a great red scarf, which made him feel a marked man, "like a dog fitted with a clog to keep him from eating the grapes." The physician and surgeon took him around the camp to visit their wounded and Ambroise kept his eyes open. He noticed that they had no more heavy artillery, but only twenty-five or thirty field pieces. Once they took him up to a prison camp near St. Omer, where a number of the French leaders were confined, to parley with M. de Baugé, brother of the late M. de Martigues. On his way back to Gravelines, Paré and his guards passed the artillery park where he saw their big siege cannon, most of them fouled and worn out. They went past Theroüenne and Hesdin, where no sign could be seen of the former fortresses, so thoroughly had the Emperor had them demolished.

M. de Vaudeville's ulcer was practically healed by this time, so, true to his word, he sent Paré to Abbeville with a guard and a passport. Hence Ambroise took the post and returned to Aufimon, where he joined the King. Henri received him cordially and called in M. de Guise, the Constable and M. d'Estrés to hear Paré's account of the fall of Hesdin. The news of the poor condition of the artillery at St. Omer was very good indeed; they had feared that the enemy might come even further into France. The King gave Paré two hundred écus to take him home and he wrote later that he was happy to be at liberty and out of the great torment and thunderous noise of the devilish artillery and far from the soldiers, "blasphemers and denyers of God." He found, too, that when the King had learned that Paré had been captured, he had had M. de Gaugier, his Premier-physician, write Madam Paré telling her that he was alive and that she should not worry, since he would pay her husband's ransom.

CHAPTER VI

Court Surgeon in a Period of Civil Strife
Two New Kings
1554-1562

BACK IN PARIS, in the summer of 1554, Paré plunged again into his old routine of writing, lecturing, dissecting and practice. Now, also, he had Court duties added to these and put in hours and days at the Louvre and at the Tournelles Palace, or on horseback, riding to one or another of the neighboring châteaus where the King might be lodged, taking his turn with the other surgeons-in-ordinary as detailed by the Premier-surgeon, in caring for the accidents and wounds suffered by the members of the King's staff. He demonstrated anatomy at the College of Surgeons, where the course became so popular that the Faculté de Médecine became alarmed over their prerogatives and the prestige of their own school. They obtained a royal decree that no more bodies were to be delivered by the authorities for dissection unless the work was done in the presence of a physician. This did not seriously interfere with the College of St. Côme; the surgeons simply put a physician in the chair to officiate and continued with their work.

His appointment as King's Surgeon-in-ordinary increased Paré's practice considerably. The manifest favor he enjoyed at the Court was embarrassing to the surgeons holding similar rank, but being less popular with His Majesty. Several of his fellow surgeons were his good friends, especially Guillaume de Bois[67] Étienne de la Rivière, who now was an official in the College of St. Côme. Rather than have a barber-surgeon hold rank equal to that of bona fide surgeons, the College decided to recruit him as a member, although this procedure was contrary to their University agreement. No doubt, de la Rivière had a guiding hand it this (Le Paulmier, p. 42 and Paget, p. 173).

On 18 August, 1554, Paré applied for permission to attempt the preliminary examination for the degree of Bachelor. On the 23rd, a Commission met informally, and most irregularly, at the home of the senior examiner, Provost le Vest,[68] and they declared M. Ambroise Paré, King's Surgeon-in-ordinary, a fit candidate for the examination. Four days later, Paré met four examiners at the Hôtel-Dieu, where they solemnly put him through the Latin examination, for which he had obviously been coached superficially. He gave feeble answers inelegantly phrased. La Rivière appealed to the examiners in his behalf. They gravely suggested that he learn more Latin and theoretical surgery, but conferred upon him the degree of Bachelor. On 1 October, Paré applied for examination for his Licentiate. A week later he was examined, sustained a disputation, and "since the King wished it," was made a Licentiate. He could now wear the Long Robe, but not the Square Hat, which was reserved for the Masters.

On 5 November, the Confraternity of St. Côme met again and agreed unanimously to make him a Master. On 3 December, Commissioners were named to assist him. These were de la Rivière, Langlois,[66] Gaignard, Ynard, Nicholas Le Brun and his son Louis, Mormorel, Du Bois, Le Gay,[70] Cheval and des Neux[71] (Le Paulmier, p. 48). On 17 December, 1554, the Confraternity and the College of St. Côme[72] met in the church of the Mathurins, which the surgeons preferred to their own of St. Jacques-de-la-Boucherie, since it was nearer the University. The Faculté was represented by Dr. Fernel and Millet. Bishops, Lords and other great people were present (Malgaigne, I, cclix). Ambroise read a Latin thesis, the subject and the translator being unknown to us. The next day he was presented to the Provost, le Vest, and received his degree of Master Surgeon of the Confraternity of St. Côme. He made his oath, recorded by Peyrilhe, although the records of the Confraternity no longer exist, and was coiffed with his Square Hat by de la Rivière. The Faculté derided the whole proceeding and twenty-three years later, when Paré was under fire by their Dean Riolan,[73] a pamphlet was published saying:

> The surgeon is to the physician what the dentist is to the surgeon—. Among surgeons who are excellent in practice, there are some (everybody knows whom I mean without my having to name them) who cannot decline their own names. We have seen them called from the barber's shop to be made Masters of Surgery, and admitted gratis against the rules, for fear the barbers, their superior skill being recognized, should put the College to shame: we have heard them declaiming in the prettiest way in the world, the Latin that someone else had breathed into them, and with no more understanding of what they said than school children set to repeat Greek speeches (Paget, p. 174).

Roilan undoubtedly was correct, technically; still, it was a battle of rules and procedures and there is no doubt that the Confraternity also was right in admitting to their ranks the foremost surgeon of the century. It was the rules that erred in being so inflexible that they had to be circumvented in order to permit a legitimate exception.

On 13 February, 1555, Jacques du Bois, or Sylvius, died in Paris in his seventy-seventh year. Always considered penurious, he was buried in the Cemetery for Poor Scholars. A little rumor circulated that when he took to his bed, he placed a pair of boots there, to be used to ford the Styx to avoid paying Charon his fee.

On 25 October, 1555, in Brussels, the Emperor Charles V, an old man of fifty-five, fat, sick and bedeviled by gout, finally made good his threat to abdicate. He made his son Philip II[74] sovereign of the Netherlands, Burgundy, Naples and the Indes. His title of Emperor went to his brother, Ferdinand, of Austria.

In 1557, war again broke out between Spain and France. In June, a Spanish army under the Duke de Savoy landed on the Channel coast and struck St. Quentin, defended by the Duke de Nevers.[75] In the battle, the old Constable had his thigh mangled by a cannon ball and was captured, as were many other French noblemen and seven thousand troops. The Prince de Condé and de Nevers fell back on La Fère with the remnants of the army.

LA FÈRE

After the battle, the King sent Paré to the Marshal de Bourdillon in La Fère for a passport to enter the Spanish camp to treat the Constable (Malgaigne, III, p. 720). La Fère, about 25 kilometers south of St. Quentin, is now a town of some 3500 people. One can see there now the house of Marie de Luxembourg, in which Paré's friend, Antoine de Bourbon, King of Navarre was born. When Paré arrived, the town was overflowing with refugees from the great battle. While his request for his passport was being sent to the Duke de Savoy, Paré treated many of the wounded. He reported (Malgaigne, II, p. 8; Hamby, p. 42) the case of a man who developed a salivary fistula after sustaining a sword thrust through the cheek. Malgaigne said this was the first such case on record. Paré mentioned also that his assistant, Rostaing de Binosc was with him, a fact he did not mention in his *Journeys*.

When the reply came from the Duke de Savoy, the request for Paré's passport was denied; the surgeon knew too much of other things than surgery; frankly, the Duke considered him a spy. On being told this, the King instructed de Bourdillon to have Paré write the information he had been given in a letter to the Constable and to have this delivered by the man who took him his fresh laundry. Although Montmorency could speak several languages, it is well known that he could not read or write. Even in his captivity, he must have had trusted attendants with him. Paré was to entrust certain things to the messenger to be delivered verbally to Montmorency. This was done and Paré requested permission to return home. The Marshal begged him to stay a few days and help treat the wounded, a request he could not refuse. The wounds were very foul after the days intervening since the battle; the mortality was terrible. Paré spoke of washing maggots out of the wounds with wine. There were no medical supplies in town and, when some were found in army wagons, they were rationed out to the surgeons, who never had enough to treat the wounded properly.

Paré was entreated to go with some of the Gentlemen to the battle field to help identify the body of M. de Bois-Dauphin, who had died in battle. They found the earth covered for half a league with the dead bodies of men and horses, all in an advanced state of putrefaction in the August heat. The cadaverous stench was unbearable. When disturbed, big blue and green flies arose in "clouds thick enough to obscure the sun." Paré believed they made the air pestilent and caused the plague.

Finally, worn out with almost fruitless work, Paré became worried over his own health and asked leave to return to the King. Malgaigne rebuked Paré for this "desertion" of battlefield service, quite unfairly, I believe. He said (Introduction, p. cclxii), "He stopped then at La Fère, occupied with treating the wounded from the battle, but already fortune had swollen his head a little; the Gentlemen wounded had returned to Paris; hardly any but soldiers remained at La Fère and the crowding was such that infection attacked all the wounds. *I tired myself greatly there,* naively said the author himself; he asked then that they have other surgeons come, and he returned to Paris." We have no other account of this episode than Paré's own. Certainly, Malgaigne's interpretation of his action was strictly out of character for Ambroise. He had unquestionably proved his devotion to duty; it is entirely probable that he did not feel physically able to carry on at that time. Other surgeons were available to handle the work load, and Ambroise had other duties more pressing than those of this refugee camp. The Marshal called for other surgeons to carry on and sent Paré home with a letter to the King, praising him for his diligence in treating the wounded. On his return, Paré found more wounded Gentlemen who had retired there, waiting for him to treat them.

Furious fighting raged through northern France, but Philip was unable to attack Paris. On 1 January, 1558, the Duke de Guise, who had abandonned a campaign in Italy after the battle of St. Quentin, struck and recaptured Calais, which had been in English hands for two hundred and fifty years. Desultory fighting continued in Picardy. Thirty miles above Amiens, Doullens (spelled Dourlan by Paré) was besieged by the enemy. Henri II sent Paré there to treat the wounded.

DOULLENS (DOURLAN)

In the back-wash of the war, Picardy was overrun by bands of marauding soldiers of several nationalities. To insure his safe passage, Paré was sent to Doullens, escorted by fifty men-at-arms under the command of a Captain Guast (Malgaigne, III, p. 722). The surgeon exchanged his beautiful little hackney mare for his servant's faster horse. He and the servant exchanged hats and cloaks to confuse their identities in case of capture, in order to permit Paré more surely to reach his destination. As they approached the castle the defenders, thinking them enemies, fired cannon at them until Captain Guast was able to signal their identity with his hat. To their great relief, the party then was admitted.

Paré mentioned the case of a Captain St. Aubin, a favorite of the Duke de Guise, who was ill with quartan fever (Malgaigne, III, p. 722; Hamby, p. 180). At the height of a fever exacerbation, he got up to go on a sally with his company. Recognizing him as a Captain, a Spaniard shot him through the neck with an arquebus. Thinking himself mortally wounded, the Captain lost his fever and it never returned. Paré dressed him, with the help of Antoine Portail,[76] a King's Surgeon-in-ordinary, who later married Jacqueline de Prime, a cousin of Ambroise's wife. He and Ambroise were closely associated thereafter.

While Paré was in this camp, an epidemic of dysentery broke out (Malgaigne, III, pp. 422 and 449; Hamby, pp. 138 and 141). Paré noticed that the victims passed large amounts of blood with their bowel movements. Curious as to the mechanism of the hemorrhages, he performed autopsies on several of the victims. In the mucosa he found little masses connected to the blood vessels; when these were squeezed, blood spurted out. He noted that M. le Grand, King's Physician-in-ordinary, also there by the King's command, saved several patients by having them drink cows' milk. He also had milk injected as enemas "to neutralize the acidity of the humors." After the enemy decamped, Paré returned home.

Worn out by the wars, France, Spain and England insured a truce on 3 April, 1559, in the Peace of Château-Cambriesis. To honor the occasion, and to cement the Peace with new family alliances, Henri betrothed his sister Marguerite to his erstwhile antagonist the Duke de Savoy, and his oldest daughter Elizabeth, Catherine's favorite, to King Philip of Spain. The weddings were to be solemnized at the Palais, but the largest and gayest parties and merrymaking occurred at the Palais des Tournelles, at the site of the present Place des Vosges.

On 15 June, the Duke d'Alva arrived with the Prince d'Orange and Count Egmont of Brussels to be proxies for their King at his marriage. On 28 June, the marriage contract was signed between Marguerite and the Duke de Savoy. On the same day began a three-day tournament to climax the nuptual festivities. On the last day of the tournament, where Henri had been a splendid performer, he insisted upon one last joust with the Count de Montgomery,[7] Captain of his Scottish Guard. The jagged butt of Montgomery's shivvered lance sprung the King's helmet visor and buried itself in his face.

Henri was helped into the Tournelles Palace and to bed. He was tough; he had lived most of his forty years in the saddle and his courage was unquestioned. With only one outcry, he endured the surgeons' extraction of five splinters from his right eye and temple. For three days he improved, while the courtiers plotted and intrigued for such advantages as they could wrest from the disaster. The King asked for Montgomery, who had fled Paris, and absolved him from any culpability in the accident. On the fifth day, Vesalius arrived from Brussels at the order of Philip, to take over the management of the case. Paré thus met the famous anatomist again, whether or not they actually became personally acquainted. Vesalius was an educated Physician and the Premier of his King; Paré still was only a surgeon, although as he wrote later to Dr. Chapelain, his advice was solicited from time to time in management of the case. Ambroise must have been intensely interested in the man whom he regarded as the Master Anatomist, since at the moment he was writing such a book himself and was having some illustrations made on the model of the Master's own.

Gradually, the severity of the injury and the action of the infection gained ascendancy over the King's burly strength and will to live. At intervals he was conscious and participated in governmental affairs, but on 10 July, after eleven agonized days, Henri II was dead. The fifteen-year-old François was King, but his powers were uncertain, since he was barely of legal age (14 years) to inherit the kingdom, and the question of a Regency was not settled. Adroitly, the Guises moved in, as relatives of the young Queen Marie,[78] and the old Constable was slipped out before he realized it. Perhaps most legally entitled to the Regency, being Princes of the Blood, the Bourbons were too tinged with Protestantism to permit their challenging the Guises easily. So François de Guise, the popular warrior and his brother Charles Cardinal de Lorraine, the suave and clever diplomat, assumed major power. To appease the Bourbons, they gave Condé the government of Picardy and put the King of Navarre and the Prince de la Roche-sur-Yon on the Council. This was not sufficient, however, and the French separated gradually into two antagonistic and armed religious factions that shortly were engaged in civil war.

The appointments of the King's Household were not made until New Year's Day, so Ambroise remained at his post of Surgeon-in-ordinary in the Court of the new young King.

On 14 July, four days after King Henri's death, Paré went to the Châtelet and made a donation of fifteen livres tournois to Olive Arnoullet, the six or seven year old daughter of M. Amy Arnoullet, Doctor of Medicine, living in Sezanne, a village near Epernay (Le Paulmier, pp. 52 & 181). This money was part of the revenue coming to Ambroise from the salt tax levied on several Norman villages. We don't know why he made the donation, beyond the statement of the bequest, "from the good friendship the said Paré held for the said M. Amy Arnoullet and in return for the good things he had done for him." It seems likely that Arnoullet had befriended him on some wearisome trip he had made into the north countries in the wars. It is probable that the friendship persisted, for in his book on

Monsters and Prodogies, Paré recorded receiving from Sezanne data on a malformed lamb born on 13 April, 1573 (Malgaigne, III, p. 45).

On 10 August, Ambroise was back in court again making a deposition in a trial that caused a great scandal. On 24 March, 1557, Françoise de Rohan, daughter of Paré's old friend, the Vicount de Rohan, had delivered out of wedlock a son whom she called Henri. She then brought suit against Jacques de Savoy, Duke de Nemours, accusing him of having seduced her on promise of marriage, but abandoning her because of Anne d'Este, wife of the Duke de Guise. Mlle. de Rohan was one of the Queen-Mother's Maids-of-Honor; in her complaint she named the Queen-Mother, Diane de Poitiers, the Constable de Montmorency and others.

Paré testified that he had known Mlle. de Rohan for ten or twelve years and that at her call he had gone to the Louvre to bleed her. At the door he was met by Dr. Joachim de Salon, the Queen-Mother's Premier-physician, who, without giving him any reason for the decision, forbade him to bleed her (Le Paulmier, p. 53). He had learned later that the Lady was pregnant by the Duke de Nemours. Mlle. de Rohan lost the suit, but always considered herself the Duke's legitimate wife and refused to marry. A year after the Duke died in 1586, she signed a marriage contract with François de Felle, Seigneur de Guebriant. The Lady herself died in December of 1591; her son Henri died five years later (Le Paulmier, p. 54).

On the day of this deposition, 10 August, 1559, Jeanne Mazelin bore Ambroise his second son, destined to live only a year. The child was baptized and christened Isaac, in St. André-des-Arts church. His godfathers were his uncle Antoine Mazelin, the court clerk whose property Ambroise had acquired, and Nicole Lambert, another of the King's Surgeons-in-ordinary. His godmother was Anne de Tillet, daughter of Seraphin de Tillet, President of the Chambers of Accounts of Paris, wife of Estienne Lallemant, Seigneur de Vouzay, King's Councillor and Master of Petitioners of the Royal House.

In December, Ambroise was listed in the *Archives* list of the servants of King François II as "Chirurgien Varlet-de-Chambre" at a salary of 240 livres, Nicole Lavernault[79] being Premier (Le Paulmier, p. 191).

1560

Ambroise's trunk-maker brother Jean had lived in the rue de la Huchette with his wife Marie de Neufville and their daughter Jeanne, her uncle's favorite. Jean Paré had died an unknown time earlier, and Ambroise and his wife took little Jeanne to live with them. On 15 January, 1560, the Paré's went before their notaries at the Châtelet and settled upon their niece the sum of five hundred livres tournois for her dowry, in case she lived to marry; otherwise the money would revert to Ambroise's estate. On 1 March, they paid over the money, to be managed by the attorneys in her interest (Le Paulmier, p. 217).

On 2 August, 1560, Paré's son Isaac, just a year old, died and was buried in the church of St. André-des-Arts. On 29 September, a daughter was born and was baptized Catherine in the same church. This was the last child born to Ambroise and Jeanne Mazelin for the remaining thirteen years of the mother's life. Her godfather was Gaspard Martin, Barber-surgeon husband of Ambroise's sister Catherine. Her godmothers were her grandmother, Jeanne de Prime, wife of Estienne Cléret; Marguerite, who became Cléret's second wife after Jeanne de Prime's death; and Catherine, wife of her cousin Loys de Prime. These godparents were all from the family (Le Paulmier, p. 56).

The young King François II had had a tempestuous year of reign. Civil war had disrupted the country and the Catholics and the Huguenots[80] were at one another's throats. On 17 November, 1560, while the King was mounting his horse for a hunt, he fainted. He took to his bed quite ill with an earache, and Paré was active in his treatment. On 30 November, the King fainted again, and his condition deteriorated. A veritable tug-of-war for influence played around the young King's bed, the Guises vs. the Bourbons. Finally, on 5 December, François II died, aged seventeen, hated throughout his kingdom. In the turmoil following so fateful an occasion, Ambroise was accused of having poisoned the King while dressing his ear, but the maliciousness of the rumor was too apparent for serious consideration. Paré was retained at his regular post by the young King Charles IX, who followed his brother François to the throne.

Charles was ten and a half years old, amiable, alert, graceful and active. Tall and thin, he was a sportsman fond of hunting, riding and tennis. Artistic, and capable in painting and sculpture, he disliked study and business. Because fourteen was the age fixed by law as that of majority of the French Kings, a Regency was necessary. Catherine had secured this for herself even before the death of François, and she took over immediately. The Guises had no legal power, now that their niece no longer was Queen, and Catherine forced a truce between them and the Bourbons. Catherine tried to conciliate everyone. As she wrote to her daughter Elizabeth, Queen of Spain, "God had left me with three young children and a kingdom divided against itself, without a soul in whom I can place the slightest confidence" (Roeder).

1561

From the heirs of Jean Mestreau, in 1561 Ambroise bought the Maison des Trois Maures, the House of the Three Moors, next door to the Maison de la Vache, moved into it and lived there until he died. The property had a large courtyard extending down to the river front; the present quais had not then been constructed. Later, upon this block of land, Ambroise gathered his friends and relatives around him.

Through all the turmoil of the Court, politics, and his busy private practice, Ambroise had continued working upon a comprehensive, illustrated textbook of anatomy, more complete than the *Brief Collection* published in 1549. Thierry de Héry had helped him with the earlier dissections, but Binosc was working at it now. Paré took this book to Jean le Royer, son of Anges Sucevin, widow of Jean de Brie, who, ten years earlier had published his book on *Gunshot Wounds*. Appointed King's Engraver in 1554, le Royer became King's Printer in 1560 (Doe, p. 49). The illustrations, and particularly the fine engraved portrait, show the Royer touch. Getting into trouble later for publishing prohibited books, le Royer fled to Geneva in 1577.

The printing of the book, *Anatomie Universelle du Corps*

Humain was finished on 15 April 1561, and made a better appearance than had Paré's earlier ones. It was pocket-sized, measuring 10 x 16 cm, and much handier for the practicing surgeon to carry than were the larger-sized ones commonly printed. It had two hundred seventy-seven pages and forty-nine woodcuts, the anatomical ones modified from those of Vesalius, to whom Paré gave credit, and the surgical ones of his own design. It is not known whether Ambroise personally prepared sketches for them, or if this was done by hired artists. While the book contained no new anatomical facts of Paré's discovery, it was designed to put the best anatomical information into the hands of those most needing it. He dedicated his book to the King of Navarre. Under his own portrait his motto, *Labor improbus omnia vincit*, "Constant work conquers everything," appeared in print for the first time. The book later was reproduced almost exactly in the first edition of his *Oeuvres* in 1575, and reappeared in Malgaigne's edition (v. I, p. 105), without the illustrations. It filled a great need and remained highly popular as a text well into the seventeenth century.

On 4 May, 1561, Ambroise sustained an injury which, at that time, must have struck sheer horror through him, since it exposed him to the possibility of crippling, the loss of a leg, or indeed, of his life. He described it in considerable detail in his book on *Fractures* (Malgaigne, II, p. 328; Hamby, p. 82).

Paré started a trip on horseback that morning with Dr. Jean Nestor,[81] Regent Physician of the Faculté de Médecine, Richard Hubert,[82] and Antoine Portail, King's Surgeons-in-ordinary, to visit some patients in the village of Bons-Hommes, near Paris. This was outside the city walls at the present location of the Chaillot Palace. Having to cross the Seine, they took a ferry that must have crossed at about the site of the present Pont d'Iena, in front of the Eiffel Tower.

In getting his horse aboard, Paré switched him. The horse kicked him in the left leg above the ankle. As Ambroise stepped back upon it ,the bones struck through the flesh, his stocking and boot, driving into the dirty floor of the boat. He fell in an agony of pain. Not being able to dress him properly in the crowded boat, his companions had the boat rowed across the river and carried him into a house. He described the pain of the trip. As the motion grated the bones and cut the flesh, he was drenched with sweat: "if I had been thrown into the water, I could not have been wetter." He was put to bed. Portail and Hubert reduced the comminuted fracture, dressed it with such things as were available for use in such places: egg whites, flour and chimney soot, with fresh melted butter and fixed it in a splint made of wicker or reeds. Knowing all too well the serious probable consequences of dirty compound fractures, and in fear of losing his leg, Paré begged M. Hubert to forget anything he might owe him in friendship and to treat him as he would any other patient with such an injury. Despite the plea, he could not refrain from offering M. Hubert a great deal of minute advice about debridement of the wound, the manual reapposition of bone fragments and the dressing. It must have been a harrowing experience for his attendants as well as for himself!

After the wound had been dressed and the leg splinted, Paré was taken back to his own house where he was bled of three palettes, about nine ounces, from the left basilic vein. His old friend, Étienne de la Rivière, took charge of him here and treated him through his illness. During each of the first nine days, he ate only a dozen Damascus plums and six morsels of bread, and drank a pint of Hippocras, which was merely sweetened, boiled water, flavored with cinnamon. He was permitted the "Divine Drink," which was nothing more than lemon-flavored, sweetened, boiled water. It may be recalled that wine was drunk regularly then, not primarily for its flavor or alcoholic content, but because water was not safe to drink. These drinks made with boiled water probably required flavoring to mask the unpleasant odors of the Seine water.

Despite this "exquisite regimen," as he termed it, Paré developed an infection, with some fever, on the eleventh day, and an abscess that drained for some time. He described the tortures of lying absolutely still upon his back, for days upon end, and the excruciating torment arising from pressure points about the ankle. Once in his sleep his leg jerked upright, redislocating the fracture and requiring its realignment, which hurt more than when it was first dressed. Finally, he reported, "It was another month before I could put the foot weakly to the ground. This was painful at first, as the callus held the tendons. While it would seem that movement should be free, the tendons and membranes must gradually be loosened from the scar." He concluded his account, "Finally, thanks to God, I was entirely healed, without limping in any way." He was back at work sometime in September. His injury prevented him from witnessing the coronation of young King Charles IX at Reims on 15 May, 1561.

Sometime during this year, Paré had an amusing experience with one of his pet aversions, fraudulent beggars (Malgaigne, III, p. 52; Hamby, p. 121). A wealthy, and not very astute, charitably minded lady called him, with Dr. Houllier and Germain Cheval,[83] to examine a poor beggar woman who had a "snake in her belly." They examined the plump, well-developed strumpet and heard her story. She was from Normandy, where she worked in the hemp fields. Once while she slept in the field, this dragon had sneaked into her interior and subsequently had made her life miserable with its writhings. She had traveled far since, gathering many alms from good ladies who were invited to put their hands upon her abdomen to feel the turmoil created by this beast. Her present benefactor was more charitable; beyond giving her financial help, she sought to have her cured of her affliction by calling eminent medical and surgical people to her assistance. They conferred. Dr. Houllier gave the patient a strong purgative. The medicine worked beautifully, but the stubborn serpent refused to come out. At another consultation they put her on a table, "displaying her ensign," as Paré reported, and he introduced a vaginal speculum, dilating her well to see if any glimpse of her boarder could be had. Failing at this, they proposed frankly to purge her continuously until her reluctant inhabitant departed. She confessed her imposture then; the writhings were voluntarily produced by her abdominal muscles, as the Doctors had suspected from the start. She left that night, taking her clothes, as well as some of those of her hostess. A week later, Paré saw her again at the gate of Montmartre, sprawled over a pack-horse, displaying her ample charms to the fish mongers with whom she was on her way home.

1562

On 28 January, 1562, Ambroise went before his lawyers at the Châtelet and ceded a portion of his courtyard to Master-Painter Guillaume Gueau and his wife Claude Périer. These were the relatives of Marie Périer, first wife of Ambroise's brother Jean, who had been so kind to Jean after Marie's death (see p. 55). This was Ambroise's chance to reciprocate. The bequest permitted Gueau to build a house facing the river and separated by a narrow alley from the house of his brother-in-law, François Périer, another Master-Painter. On the East, the Gueau house adjoined that of Charles de Paris, Master-Pastry Cook. Ambroise specified that the Gueau house should be built no higher than the Périer house, permitting him to have a view of the city over their roof-tops from the upper windows of his own houses across the courtyard. The erection of this new house and the placing of a stout gate between it and the Périer house completed the enclosure of Paré's courtyard, isolating it from the riverfront traffic and from the constantly increasing street strife incidental to the civil unrest. Paré gave the house to the Gueaus to use and enjoy during their lifetimes, but its ownership remained with him and his heirs.

Since the death of King Henri, Dr. Chapelain[84] had been urging Paré to write a book on *Head Injuries*. The anatomical portion was already prepared, derived from his *Anatomie Universelle*. Ambroise probably worked upon this while immobilized by his broken leg. He wrote up the case reports and added the material on surgical management. Illustrations were prepared of the instruments required, since they were not available elsewhere, and several were of Paré's own invention. He acknowledged his debt to Vesalius for the models of some of his anatomical figures. A woodcut portrait done by Jean Cousin was printed in an oval surrounded by his motto, *Labor improbus omnia vincit*. This was reprinted, with the age changed from forty-five to fifty-five, in his *Five Books of Surgery* in 1572. Ambroise dedicated the book to M. Chapelain, and said that the manuscript had been read by Dr. Robert Greaume, a member of the Faculté, who had furnished the Greek terms Paré used.

This book, with two hundred seventy-six pages of text and seventy-four woodcuts, finished printing on 28 February, 1561/62, and appeared under the title: *La Méthode Curative des Playes, & Fractures de la Teste Humain. With the pictures of the Instruments necessary for the cure of such.* By M. Ambroise Paré Ordinary Surgeon of the King & Sworn at Paris. At Paris. From the Press of Jean le Royer, King's Printer in Mathematics, in the rue St. Jacques, at the sign of the True Potter, near the Mathurins, With King's Privilege. 1561.

The book's date of appearance has raised some modern questions (Doe, p. 52), since Ambroise called himself Ordinary Surgeon, and not Premier, which he became on New Year's Day, 1562. Le Paulmier, p. 57, dated the ceremony on 1 January 1562, wondering why Paré had not used his new title in this book. Malgaigne (Intro., cclxviii) had no precise date for the promotion. This confusion again was caused by the method used then for calculating the onset of the year; 28 February, 1561/62, is in 1562 by the new calendar, but not by the old. New Year's Day of 1562 had not yet come, and 28 February still belonged to 1561. While the *Anatomie Universelle* of April 1561 was already out for ten months, this new one of 28 February, 1561/62, was only now going before the public.

CHAPTER VII

Ambroise Paré, King's Premier-Surgeon
1562-1564

On New Year's Day, 1562, which was on Easter, members of the King's Household gathered, as was the custom, at St. Germain-en-Laye to renew their oaths of allegiance to the King and to have their commissions renewed. The splendid château at St. Germain, on the left bank of the first northern loop of the Seine beyond Paris, was a favorite residence of the Royal Family. Kings Henri II and Charles IX were born there. Rebuilt by François I, only the donjon of Charles V and the Châpelle of St. Louis had been retained from the past ages. The château and its grounds remain as impressive relics of the architectural ambitions of the earlier Kings. The Châpelle was built in 1238, a dozen years earlier than the Sainte-Châpelle in Paris and by the same architect, Pierre de Montreuil.

In this beautiful setting, the physicians were sworn in. Then the surgeons filed before the King's Councilor and Maitre-d'Hôtel, the Duke de Mendoce. They had no Premier or Chief to head their ranks, M. Nicole Lavernault having died in the past year. Ambroise was appointed King's Premier-Surgeon. His staff included, among others, his friends de la Rivière, Laurent Colot,[85] and Jacques Guillemeau.[86] Paré had been in the Court during almost the entire lifetime of the young King, to whom he was a great friend and favorite. This new post laid upon Ambroise's shoulders new responsibilities and many duties requiring more of his time and energies in attendance at the Court.

Early in this year, the Catholics and Huguenots grasped some of the numerous examples of religious strife as reasons for formal conflict and the First War of Religion burst into flame. The Huguenots, under the able leadership of Condé and Coligny, obtained English assistance. Catherine was forced to oppose them and organized her armies under the command of François de Guise. Antoine de Bourbon, King of Navarre, cast his lot against his brothers and led one of the King's armies to Bourges.

BOURGES

Paré made his first trip with the King's army against the Huguenots to Bourges, where, after a short siege, the city capitulated. Paré told (Malgaigne, III, p. 732; Hamby, p. 189) of a silly kitchen boy who, looking up at the city walls, shouted, "Huguenot, Huguenot, Shoot here! Shoot here!" One of them obliged him indeed, shooting him through the hand. As he came weeping to Ambroise to dress him, the Constable saw him and asked what had happened. A Gentleman who had witnessed the incident described it. The Constable told the lad that the Huguenot was a fine shot and a good fellow, for, had he wished, he could have shot him through the head even more easily. Paré dressed the luckless boy, who recovered with a crippled hand and the nickname of "Huguenot," which he bore thereafter.

Condé retreated to Rouen, where the garrison was reinforced by five hundred Englishmen in command of Gabriel de Montgomery, who had accidently killed Henri II. Although the dying King forgave him, Catherine never did, and Montgomery had fled to England. There he became Protestant and subsequently a Huguenot leader. The King's army of eighteen thousand men marched on Rouen under the command of the King of Navarre in October and invested the city for a siege.

ROUEN

The King of Navarre was inspecting the defenses on horseback when he was shot in the shoulder by a sniper. He was dressed by his surgeon, M. Gilbert, "one of the best of Montpellier," and others; they could not find the bullet. Ambroise, called in (Malgaigne, III, p. 723; Hamby, p. 181), also searched for it diligently. He found that it had struck the top of the humerus. Since there was no wound of exit, he concluded that it had run down the marrow cavity of the bone. Others thought it had gone into the chest. The Prince de la Roche-sur-Yon, Paré's old friend, inquired privately of him if the wound was mortal. Since the Prince loved the King, Paré told him that in his opinion it was, as were most severely contused wounds of major joints. Other surgeons and physicians were more hopeful, an opinion which pleased the patient's friends. Four days later, the King, the Queen-Mother, the Prince de la Roche-sur-Yon, the Cardinal de Bourbon, the patient's brother, and a number of other notables came to see the wound dressed. Thereafter, they assembled the physicians and surgeons and demanded a consultation in their presence. All the consultants except Paré offered a favorable prognosis. Roche-sur-Yon drew Paré aside and asked him not to be obstinate against the opinions of so many good men, since he was very fond of Ambroise and disliked seeing him in a bad position. Paré told him that he must hold that opinion until good evidence of improvement gave him a chance to change it. Although many consultations were held, the arm gradually became gangrenous, as Paré had predicted, and on the eighteenth day, the forty-four year old King of Navarre died.

The Prince de la Roche-sur-Yon wanted the bullet, perhaps to give Paré a chance to prove his diagnosis. Since he was the patient's cousin, he sent the surgeon le Fèvre[87] to Paré, instructing him to find the ball and to send it to him. Ambroise was glad to have the opportunity. He found the bullet in the cavity of the humerus near its head, as he had predicted. He sent it to the Prince, who showed it to the King and the Queen-Mother, who were duly impressed. The King's body was interred at the Château-Gaillard, the old fortress on the Seine built by Richard the Lion-Hearted at Les Andelys in 1203.

Before the King of Navarre died, Rouen fell on 26 October. For eight days the victors sacked the city. Condé escaped and rejoined the Huguenot armies. Paré worked hard with the wounded, but many patients died, both within and without the city, each side believing the other had poisoned its bullets. Infection had never much impressed the leaders before, when only common soldiers died in great numbers, but now the nobles were as vulnerable to the rapidly growing hails of bullets as were the villiens, and the mortality became a terrible concern.

Paré trepanned eight or nine men whose skulls had been fractured by stones at the breach in the city walls. He reported (Malgaigne, II, p. 22; Hamby, p. 25) showing M. Chapelain, King's Premier-Physician and M. Castellan,[88] Premier-Physician of the Queen, the case of a Gentleman whose brain was lacerated by fragments indriven from the inner table of the skull, while the outer table remained intact.

Paré returned to Paris then, where he remained very busy caring for casualties of the battle who also had returned to the city for treatment. He noted especially that these included many Italians, who had probably been sent to Catherine's assistance. There he found also that his friend and collaborator, Rostaing de Binosc, had died during his absence, on 17 October. The city was in the throes of an epidemic of plague; twenty-five thousand Parisians died of it during the year. Virulent small-pox added to the misery; the seven-year-old Duke d'Alençon (Herculé, the King's youngest brother) was scarred badly by it.

Either on his way home from Rouen or after his arrival, Paré came near death by poisoning (Malgaigne, III, p. 662; Hamby, p. 153). He recorded that he was at dinner with a group "including some who hated me to the death for the Religion." He was served some cabbage. The first bite went unnoticed. With the second, he felt in his mouth and throat the burn and astringence of a poison, and tasted the "flavor of the good drug" that he suspected was arsenic or sublimate. He immediately washed his mouth with wine and water, and drank a large quantity of it. Going to the house of the nearest apothecary, he vomited. He drank a pint of oil, retained it for a while, and vomited that. Then he drank a large amount of milk and butter and a couple of egg yolks; this ended the hazard. He remarked dryly that he never again ate cabbage, or anything else, in that company.

Paré's remark about being hated "for the Religion," and other small scattered remarks, have been accepted by many as a profession of Huguenotism, since this was a common designation of their faith. Le Paulmier (p. 80) stated flatly that Paré had so declared himself in a note made during his controversy with the Faculté in 1575 and reprinted (p. 222) the entire memoir. On page 243, item 24 reads:

> In this story which I told of myself on page 939, I have written so that one poisoned could help himself by means of such remedies. However, my enemies have maliciously tried to interpret this word of Religion so as to incite against me the hatred of all good people. It was cited, not to glorify myself as having followed such an opinion, but for fear the reader would think the attempt was made on my life in reprisal for some crime I had committed against someone's life or property. It was written even less to suggest that those following the Holy Roman Catholic Church used illegal means of disposing of their enemies. I hereby declare that such poisoners are neither of one religion or the other, but simply libertines having no fear of God.

I cannot follow Le Paulmier in his interpretation of this statement. To me it seems a model of ambiguity, purposely designed to leave himself in a neutral position, giving offense to neither side of the controversy. He served the Bourbons as faithfully as he did the Guises and the Valois, but he retained his affiliation with the Catholic Church of his parish, St. André-des-Arts, throughout his life and stood godfather to children of his Catholic friends in his old age.[89] It seems highly unlikely that, at the time especially, the Church would have permitted assumption of such a role by even a mildly suspected heretic. Doe cited Paré's employment of Huguenot printers in producing his books, when there were plenty of Catholic publishers to be had. Paré's entire record is one of intense loyalty to his personal friends; all his publishers were his near neighbors. It seems improbable that he would have selected them deliberately on the basis of their faiths. He probably would have chosen to help especially those who were having a hard time for any reason. The suspicion has remained, however, and it is the rare modern historian who does not refer to him as "the Huguenot surgeon of the Catholic French Court."

After the fall of Rouen, the Huguenots struck at Paris, but

fell afoul of Guise's Royal army at Dreux. There, on 19 December, 1562, a great battle was fought. It was costly to both sides in lives of able leaders and in the wounding and capture of others. The latter condition befell the Constable, of the victorious Royalists, and Condé of the Huguenots. Coligny took over Huguenot leadership and retreated to Orléans; Guise pursued and invested the city.

DREUX

The day after the battle of Dreux, the King sent Paré to treat the Count d'Eu (Malgaigne, III, p. 724; Hamby, p. 182). On the morning of the battle, he had been wounded by a pistol shot fired accidentally by M. de Bordes, one of his own Gentlemen. Paré found the head of the femur splintered by the ball and, to Paré's great sorrow, the Count died within a few days.

On the day after his arrival, Paré visited the battlefield and found it covered for a league around with bodies of men killed within two hours of furious fighting. He said that they were estimated to number twenty-five thousand, but historians put the figure at nearer seven thousand, approximately twenty-nine thousand combattants having participated. Even at the reduced figure, a quarter of those engaged died; the wounded were even more numerous. Paré treated a great many of them. He recalled treating fourteen gunshot victims in a single room; they all recovered. Other surgeons came from Paris to treat the wounded, including Paré's friends Pigray,[90] Cointeret,[91] and Hubert. After the death of M. d'Eu, Paré did not remain long at Dreux, but returned to Paris where many of the survivors of the battle had retired to be treated, and he dressed many of them.

Ambroise reported (Malgaigne, II, p. 613; Hamby, p. 99) treating one of the Constable's Gentlemen who had suffered severance by a cutlass stroke of the extensor tendons of the right thumb. After the wound healed, the thumb remained flexed in the palm, so he could not open the hand without lifting the thumb with the opposite hand. This made it impossible for him to hold a sword, dagger, lance or other instrument of his sole trade, which was warfare. He thus became an actual total casualty. He asked Paré to amputate the thumb. Since this also would leave the hand incapable of grasping, Paré advised against it. He had a tin appliance made for him, with rings and lanyards that let the thumb be extended, putting the Gentleman back to work at the profession of his choice and training.

On 18 February, 1563, the Catholics lost their ablest General and France a great son. While riding home in the evening from the camp where he directed the siege of Orléans, François Duke de Guise was ambushed and assassinated by Jean Poltrot, a petty nobleman of Méré, a zealot and a mercurial soldier-of-fortune. The murderer was captured two days later by Swiss soldiers. Under torture, he confessed his crime and named Coligny and other Huguenot leaders as his instigators. While Coligny was able to clear himself in the Council, he never convinced the Guises, who pursued him relentlessly until his death. Poltrot was tried, convicted and sentenced to the fate of regicides. On 18 March, he was hanged and quartered in the Place-de-Greve, before the Hôtel-de-Ville of Paris.

Catherine then was able to bring the captives, Montmorency and Condé, together to plan a truce. On 19 March, the "Edict of Amboise" was proclaimed. All religious prisoners were freed. Religion was to be recognized locally according to the church of greatest strength; the Huguenots were excluded from public office and their religion was forbidden in Paris. Condé was unhappy over the final form of the peace and the Catholics were no more joyful, but it was a necessary momentary step. The country was in a terrible state and needed time to recover. The First war of Religion was over.

On the death of the King of Navarre, the Prince de Condé was the senior Prince-of-the-Blood and, as such, was entitled to be Regent or Lieutenant-General of France. This the Catholics could not tolerate, so the twelve-year-old King Charles IX was declared of age and competent to rule. The Guises, the Montmorencies, the Bourbons and the Châtillons laid down their arms and worked together to renovate the country. United again, they needed a common foe to weld them together. Catherine sent a combined army against the English at Le Havre. The town was poorly defended and, after a six-day siege, capitulated on 28 July 1563.

LE HAVRE

Paré reported briefly on that campaign (Malgaigne, III, p. 722). He attributed the easy victory to the plague that had been raging in the city. The King permitted the defenders to take their valuables and to sail away to England. They took the plague with them and, as Paré remarked, England had not been free of it since; he was not aware that the plague had been in England too since the 12th century.

Ambroise was busy writing another book on surgery. Rumors were circulating in Paris that Paré's method of treating wounds was responsible for the high mortality rate among the wounded at Rouen. Catherine and the King asked him about it and advised him to make a statement. In his new book he discussed, all over again, the matter of the supposed poisonous character of gunshot wounds. He noted that gunpowder could be swallowed or put into an open wound without ill effect. He argued that the infection must be introduced into the wound from its surroundings, possibly from the air itself, an advanced idea in an epoch antedating bacteriology.

CHAPTER VIII

Court Tour of France with Charles IX
1564-1566

1564

In January of 1564, Catherine decided to get out of Paris and away from the intrigues between the rival factions. She gave as her reasons the desirability of becoming more intimately acquainted with the peoples and the resources of the country. Moreover, she would take a leaf from the book of her illustrious old father-in-law, François I, and give an intimate glimpse of the Court and of their young kings to the people who never had a chance to see them. While François had traveled with a retinue that often required twelve thousand horses, she planned on a more modest scale, only eight hundred of them. Preparations were made for a real traveling circus.

In the Bibliothèque Nationale can be found a small day-to-day diary of the Court journey, written by Abel Jouan, Somier (person in charge of equipment) of the King's kitchen. The five-year privilege of printing was given at St. Mordes on 10 May 1566. Le Gras wrote a more romantic, but probably less factual account of the trip, and the report by Chaussade is quite sketchy. Jouan told where the King dined each day, where he slept and the distance traveled. The daily trips covered from one to eleven leagues, usually only three to five. The league was an old European measure of distance adopted by the Romans from the Gauls, equivalent to 1500 Roman paces, or roughly one and a half miles. The distances Jouan listed were probably broad guesses, for in some instances where the distances are known, his estimates are difficult to justify by any formula. Considering the duration and the importance of the journey, surprisingly little has been written about it by general historians that I have read.

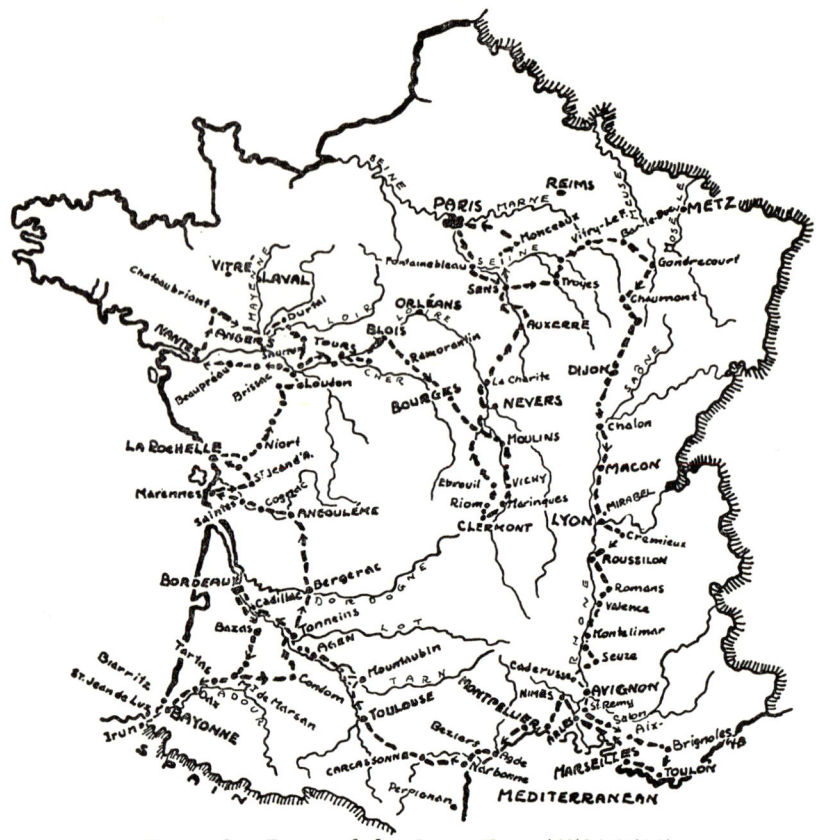

Figure 9. Route of the Court Tour (1564-1566).

Jouan reported that the Court left Paris on Monday, 24 January 1563, old reckoning, or 1564 by the new, going two leagues to St. Mordes, "a pretty village, château and abbey," where they remained for six days. On Sunday, 30 January, they crossed the Marne bridge at Charenton to Ville-Neuf-St. George, then over the Seine bridge to Corbeil, "a pretty village," where they slept—7 leagues.

On Monday, 31 January, the entourage reached Fontainebleau (8 leagues), where the travelers remained for forty-three days preparing for the long journey. Jouan recorded that they kept Lent there. On the Sunday before "Dimanche Gras" (Shrove Sunday), M. le Constable gave a dinner. On "Jeudi Gras"

(Shrove Thursday), M. le Cardinal de Bourbon gave a supper, after which the guests were entertained by a combat on horses. On Dimanche Gras, M. de Retz (son of the Marshal d'Annebault, who succeeded Paré's first military chief, M. de Montejan, as Governor of Piedmont) and the Count de Ringrave fenced. On Mardi Gras the King gave a dinner at the Hermitage; this was followed by a theatre and a combat.

Paré must have anticipated the trip with some annoyance. His book was in press, and naturally he must have feared a conflict of dates. Malgaigne (Intro., p. cclxxi) implied that the book was published while Paré was away from Paris. Apparently, he did not realize that the Court remained at Fontainebleau for two and a half months. This permitted Paré to spend all the time required in Paris. Fortunately, all came off well. Printing was finished on 3 February, 1564, new calendar, with privileges of printing granted to Paré for nine years. It was entitled *Dix Livres de la Chirurgie, avec Le Magasin des Instrumens necessaires à icelle,* or *Ten Books of Surgery, with the Stock of Necessary Instruments.* It contained forty-four leaves and two hundred thirty-two pages of print, with one hundred fifty-eight wood-cut illustrations. The title-page was designed by Jean Cousin and presumably was engraved by Jean le Royer King's Engraver and Printer (Doe, p. 53).

This, Paré's most ambitious book to date, was dedicated to the King. It contained a careful revision and rewriting of the second edition of the book on *Gunshot Wounds* and added three chapters on Urology, borrowed largely from Thierry de Héry, Pierre Franco,[92] Jacques Roy and Laurent Colot. Unfortunately, Ambroise did not credit these authors, but he corrected the omission in the 1575 edition of his *Oeuvres*. In this book, he first described hemostasis in amputations, by ligatures instead of the cautery, a technique which he had first accomplished at Damvilliers. Here, he printed his views on the high infectious rate among the wounded at Rouen. Here, too, he described the account of the compound fracture of his own ankle. It was a distinguished book for the period and one of which he justly could be proud.

On 13 March, 1564, the Court left Fontainebleau, the personnel reduced—for economy's sake—to eight hundred people. The Court included among others, Condé, the Constable, Chancellor l'Hôpital, Coligny, the Cardinals de Guise and de Loraine, the Duke de Montpensier, the Marshal de Bourdillon and the Prince de la Roche-sur-Yon. Beside the King and the Queen-Mother went her next son Henri, Duke d'Orléans; the ten-year-old François, Duke d'Anjou; Henri de Navarre and Henri de Guise, François' son. This younger generation was to figure largely in the political and military history of the next forty years. There were four companies of men-at-arms, a company of light-horse, a regiment of French Guards and hundreds of lackeys, cooks, grooms and menials. Large groups of important people would join the entourage at various places, travel with the Court for some days, then return to their own affairs. The medical attendants included Drs. Chapelain and Castellan and Ambroise, among others. The great company filled the roads, traveling on horseback, in coaches, carts and litters, and on foot. To carry her voluminous material of correspondence, since she was an indefatiguable letter-writer, Catherine went by litter. A splendid equestrienne, she probably rode horseback a great deal, using the new side-saddle she had invented. She was getting fat now, and a change of accommodation would be pleasant.

On that first day after dinner, which was eaten late in the morning, the tour got under way and the company traveled five leagues, reaching Montereau-sur-Yonne, "a little village and château where the Yonne falls into the Seine," and there they slept. At first, the way led eastward, via Sens to Troyes, then by Arcis to Vitry-le-François and on to Bar-le-Duc, where the Tour arrived on the first of May. Here lived Catherine's daughter Claude, married to Charles the Grand, Duke de Lorraine. The journey was interrupted there for a week, to permit Catherine to help christen a new grandchild.

Paré was on the alert for surgically interesting topics and he reported several of them later. In Vitry-le-François (Malgaigne, III, p. 19; Hamby, p. 110) he saw a well proportioned, heavy-bearded man named Germain Garnier, whom some also called Germain Marie, for "Marie" had been considered a girl until he was fifteen years old. "She" had looked and acted like a normal girl in all respects until one day, while out in the field vigorously chasing some pigs, she suddenly had to jump a ditch. She jumped and immediately and painlessly developed the genitalia of a man. Paré supposed that this was due to the rupture of some ligaments that earlier had retained these parts. "Marie" went sobbing home to report to her mother that her entrails were coming out. Quite astonished at what she saw, the good woman called the priest and the doctor. They examined the child and pronounced Marie a boy. The Bishop assembled the villagers and certified that Marie was a man. His name was changed to Germain Garnier. When Paré described the case in 1579, Germain was still living as a normal man. Packard (p. 33) found a similar story in Montaigne's essays. Montaigne had seen Germain and reported that the girls of the town sang a song warning one another not to strain too hard in jumping or running, and to keep their legs together, lest they too be turned into boys, à la Germain Marie. Such coincidental reporting might suggest that Montaigne too was on this trip, although Paré never had occasion to mention him.

While in Bar-le-Duc, Paré met Nicolas Picart, an ingenious bone-setter and surgeon of the Duke de Lorraine. In his book on *Luxations* (Malgaigne, II, p. 374), Paré reported Picart's method of reducing dislocations of the shoulder. With the patient standing on a stool beside an upright ladder, the arm was brought over a rung of the ladder so this rested in the axilla. The wrist then was bound down to a lower rung and the stool was pulled from beneath the patient's feet, snapping the head of the humerus into its socket. Picart also had various leverage devices made to accomplish such reductions less drastically. Ambroise must have enjoyed and respected Picart, for he looked him up again when he returned to Nancy in 1575 to help treat the Duchesse de Lorraine in her fatal illness.

The journey then was continued southward through Burgundy. Once famous for its fertility and wealth, this country now was in a sad state from the rigors of war, abandoned to weeds and erosion. Bands of vagabonds roamed the countryside, curiously eyeing this group of elegant vagrants so far from home. The gentry did its best to put on a good show. At strategic spots, gaily dressed nymphs danced out of rocky glens to brighten the way of the travelers, or shepherds appeared to recite long Latin poems. Fireworks would suddenly blaze in the evening skies to bemuse the weary wanderers. These side-shows could not mask the misery the land had suffered from the wars. Although the details were known from the statistics available to the Court, their bleak actuality was a depressing experience.

At Dijon on Sunday, 22 May, the Governor of Burgundy, Gaspard de Saulx, Seigneur de Tavannes, made a colorful entrance to his capital to welcome his guests in proper style. The huge ducal palace was a welcome haven after the weeks of camping, and the guests remained for four days.

From Dijon, they traveled down the famous Côte-d'Or, the thirty mile strip of hillside where grow the grapes that make the name Burgundy famous to the wine lovers of the world. Unhurriedly, they coursed this valley, and from Châlons they boated down the Saône to Mâcon. They rested here for almost a week; on the thirteenth of June they made their entry into Lyon. Paré had been here before, when he had ridden down with the Duke de Rohan on their way to the siege of Perpignan in 1542 (Malgaigne, II, p. 500; Hamby, pp. 59, 93, 165). It probably was on this visit to Lyon that Paré first met the surgeon Dalechamps, who in 1570 published his *French Surgery*. In this traditional compilation of Paul of Aegina, Celsus, Hippocrates, Galen and the Arabs, he listed Paré as the modern authority, and used his illustrations in his text (Malgaigne, Intro., p. cclxxv).

Lyon was suffering a hard plague epidemic, and Paré studied the disease under new circumstances with Doctors Castellan and Chapelain. He heard of and recorded stories of patients struck down in the midst of their regular activities, falling dead suddenly in the streets and churches (Malgaigne, III, p. 388; Hamby, p. 136. He described (Malgaigne, III, p. 458; Hamby, p. 141) how criminals took advantage of the civil turmoil to enrich themselves. A perfectly healthy visitor would be set upon by these mobsters and carried away by force. When the luckless victim cried out for help, the onlookers were assured that the man was mad with the plague and didn't know what he was saying. Taking their victim to the Hôtel-Dieu, the criminals would strip him of his valuables and deposit him under restraint into bed with the plague victims. Here he would soon become infected and die, either of frustration or of the disease.

Ambroise cited (Malgaigne, III, p. 460; Hamby, p. 142) the case of Amy Basten, widow of a Lyon surgeon who had died of the plague. Six days after his death, she fell into a dreamy state, then into a frenzy. She went to a window, tormenting her baby in her arms. To the horror of the spectators below who tried to divert her, begging her to be careful of the baby, she hurled the infant to the ground and leaped after him; both of them died.

Paré visited the local physicians and surgeons, asking about their manner of treating the plague. He asked the effect of bleeding upon the disease. He was told that the mortality was much higher among patients so treated. The answer was the same for those who were purged. Nothing seemed to have any specific beneficial effect.

The horrible stories and the grim sights of the stricken city were terribly depressing; fear of personal infection impelled the visitors to depart. On 9 July, the tour resumed, going eastward to visit Crémieux, where the King remained for seven days. On the seventeenth they arrived at Roussillon, a lovely château twenty-five kilometers south of Vienne, where they stayed for twenty-nine days. Here, Catherine conferred with the local leaders and sought a formula by which the two religions could live together in peace. Here, over the signature of the King, she issued the Edict of Roussillon, calling upon the two parties to respect one anothers religion. Nevertheless, the old fires smouldered and threatened to burst into flames. Here, too, Charles IX signed the Edict permanently establishing the First of January as New Year's Day in France.

Finally, Mlle. la Mare, one of the Queen's Ladies-in-waiting, fell ill with the plague (Malgaigne, III, p. 388; Hamby, p. 136) and developed a bubo in her groin. This subsided so that on the third day she was up and around, mentally clear and feeling well except for a little difficulty in voiding. "Nevertheless," as

Ambroise said, "on the same day she gave up her spirit to God, which is the reason we promptly left that place."

On 15 August, the Tour got under way, going down toward Provence. Nearing the Mediterranean, Catherine's spirits lifted somewhat, as if the climate of her youth restored her. On 22 August, they reached Valence, where they rested and explored for twelve days. In easy stages and with little side trips, they made their way down the Rhone valley to Mondragon, Mornas and Caderouse. For some reason, they missed the gem city of Orange, but reached Avignon on 23 September. Jouan wrote of the magnificent entry the King made into the city. In a huge new theatre built in the great Court before the Cathedral, the Papal Legate received them and granted absolution to all in the party. The visitors tarried here until 16 October, when they went on to St. Rémy, then to Touret and to Salon.

Both Le Gras and d'Eschevannes wrote romantic tales of a meeting Catherine contrived between Paré and her old astrologer, Nostradamus,[93] who, after a very profitable sojourn in the French Court, had retired to Salon, a lovely town between Arles and Aix-en-Provence. A confirmed believer in astrology, Catherine is reputed to have asked Paré's opinion of it. Apparently, not wanting to get into an argument with the Queen, whose mind was not only made up, but was absolutely fixed, on the subject, he replied to the effect that this was a field too far removed from his experience for him to have a worthwhile opinion. Certainly, Paré had a touch of the prevalent reverence for the occult. He believed in witches and devils; even the Bible contained stories of them. On one occasion he wrote (Malgaigne, III, p. 61; Hamby, p. 123):

> Not long ago, in the presence of King Charles IX and Messrs. le Mareschal de Montmorency, de Rets, the Seigneur de Laussac, M. de Mazille,[94] King's Premier-Physician (which dates it after 1570, as Mazille became Premier after Chapelain's death in 1569) and M. de St. Pris, King's Valet-de-Chambre, I saw things done by an imposter and enchanter that are impossible for men to do without the help of the Devil. These deceived our sight and made false and fantastic things appear to us. The imposter confessed freely to the King that he did

these things with the assistance of a spirit to whom he was bound for three more years and who tormented him greatly. He promised that when his time was served he would be a good man. God forgive him, for it is written, 'Thou shalt not suffer a witch to live.' King Saul was cruelly punished for having talked with the witch. Moses similarly commanded the Hebrews to take pains to exterminate all enchanters.

Ambroise did not comment upon the King's failure to comply with these divine admonitions. Again he wrote (Malgaigne, III, p. 65; Hamby, p. 123), "I have seen a man who could stop bleeding from any part of the body by saying words unknown to me."

In Paré's day, so much was unknown of the physical laws now considered elementary, it was impossible for him to have escaped a degree of the popular credulity. The wonder is that he was so level-headed as to have been as little impressed as he was. Fernel required ten years to rid himself of an obsession with astrology.

From Salon, the Court continued on to Aix-en-Provence, Toulon and Marseilles, thence to Arles and to Montpellier. They made a Grand Entry into the old university city on Saturday, 17 December. The King like it so well that they sojourned there for two weeks, enjoying Christmas week. The medical school here had been the foremost of the world a century earlier, and here Paré's surgical hero, Guy de Chauliac, "le bon Guidon," had practiced and taught. Doctors Chapelain and Castellan had graduated here and, as the three were good friends, they must have "done the town" together.

Here, Ambroise met the surgeon Cabrol and Professor Joubert, who later became Chancellor of the University. In 1570, Joubert wrote a *Treatise on Arquebusades,* in the preface of which he said, "M. Ambroise Paré, the very expert and learned surgeon of the King, supports me with his immortal writings" (Malgaigne, Intro., p. cclxxv).

Paré was interested in the preparation of theriac, a complicated compound, that he and other medical people used in serious cases. He recorded at least three formulas for its preparation (Malgaigne, II, p. 599-600 and III, p. 368). Among other things, its contents included the flesh and venom of vipers. When Paré visited the apothecary named de Farges (Malgaigne, III, p. 314; Hamby, p. 129) to have an ointment of theriac made, he asked to see the snakes. He was shown a number of them kept in a glass jar and, wanting to see the fangs through which the venom is injected, he picked one of them up. The snake struck the end of his index finger between the nail and the tip. Paré reported the immediate severe pain he felt. He promptly bound the finger tightly to encourage bleeding. He had one of the apothecary's servants mix some old theriac and brandy in the palm of his hand. Ambroise dipped cotton into the mixture and held it upon the wound, which healed within a few days without more trouble.

On 30 December, 1564, the great entourage left Montpellier and crawled over the mountainous, ice-covered roads to Carcassonne, where the weary travelers rested and were entertained for two weeks. They went then to Toulouse, then by barge down the river Garonne, finally arriving at Bordeaux on Saturday, 1 April 1565.

While the notables were occupied with politics, Ambroise was busy with his surgical duties and was called into consultations in the area. On one occasion (Malgaigne, III, p. 211; Hamby, p. 123), a local physician, M. de la Taste, called him, with Drs. Chapelain and Castellan and the King's surgeon, Nicole Lambert, to examine and advise treatment for a forty-year-old Lady. She had a tumor the size of a pea situated just outside and below the left hip joint. Intermittently, she had suffered such excruciating pain in the area that all manner of treatments had been used unsuccessfully by many physicians and surgeons, as well as "wizards and witches."

Intrigued by the story, Ambroise wanted to witness one of these paroxysms, and got M. de la Taste to take him to the Lady's house. Conveniently, a pain struck her while they were there, and Ambroise recorded the "incredible movements" she demonstrated. She threw herself about, putting her head between her legs and her feet on her shoulders, with many other "marvelous movements" that continued for almost fifteen minutes. During the time, Paré was handling the area trying to discover any signs of swelling or inflammation, but the only result was louder lamentations. Finally exhausted, she fell weak and relaxed, hot and perspiring copiously. Neither Paré nor Dr. de la Taste could understand it, but they ruled out epilepsy, since such a convulsion should have left her unconscious, whereas she spoke easily and cerebrated well.

They told the story to Drs. Chapelain and Castellan, who also were amazed. They decided to apply the "potential cautery" to the tumor. After the caustic had produced its necrosis and the crust came away, a "very dark, virulent material drained and she never had another pain." Ambroise tried to fit the experience into the prevalent humeral theories of disease and finally wrote it up in his book in the section on gout. Now-a-days, the Lady probably would have been called hysterical.

The Court remained at Bordeaux through most of April, celebrating Easter there in the Cathedral with great ceremony on 22 April. The rains ceased and spring burst warmly over the land. Catherine had an appointment to meet her daughter Elizabeth, Queen of Spain, at Bayonne and to give their ministers the opportunity for a state meeting, which had to do principally with the religious question. While the ministers of the two countries conferred and jockeyed for prestige of their respective Courts in the traditional manner, the French party slowly advanced toward Bayonne. They took most of the month to get there, while the heat increased almost unbearably. They finally entered Bayonne on Thursday, 29 May. The negotiations extended through June and into early July, finally ending in a stalemate. The Spaniards insisted that Catherine and the French Government enter a crusade of annihilation of the Huguenots, which they would not do.

While the political activities were transpiring, Paré had enough to do to keep him busy. A Spanish Gentleman (Malgaigne, III, p. 733; Hamby, p. 190) came to the King begging to be touched for the scrofula, since the touch of a King was supposed to be a magic cure for the disease. Jouan tells us that this occurred on 9 June, at the Feast of the Pentecost, at Thoulouzette. Paré saw the Gentleman and diagnosed an abscess of the neck. He drained it and proved the diagnosis. The

Spaniard then revealed that he had a mass under his tongue interfering with his speech and swallowing. Encouraged by Paré's success with his neck, he asked him to operate upon this mass also, if it could be done without danger to his life. Ambroise promptly opened this ranula and found the salivary duct obstructed by five stones ranging in size from that of a small pea to an almond, with a cyst containing four teaspoonsful of liquid.

M. de la Fontaine, one of the King's Chevaliers (Malgaigne, III, pp. 734 & 419; Hamby, pp. 138 & 191), had a high, continuous, pestilential fever and many carbuncles all over his body. He developed a severe nose-bleed that could not be controlled, and which continued for ten days. The fever then abated with a profuse sweat; the bleeding ceased; the carbuncles drained and, "He was dressed by me and cured by the grace of God."

When Catherine and the Court went to St. Jean-de-Luz and left the Huguenot courtiers at Bayonne, the Prince de la Roche-sur-Yon went off to Biarritz to nurse a headache that had been tormenting him constantly for some time. Despite the treatment of the Court physicians, he got no better. Finally, the Prince asked Dr. Loys Duret, who visited him frequently in Biarritz, to bring Paré to see him. Paré loved the old gentleman and rode over with the physicians to "the little village of Biarritz" (Malgaigne, II, p. 411; Hamby, p. 88) to see him. Since nothing else had helped, Ambroise advised the Prince to have the temporal artery opened on the side of the greatest pain. He had done this successfully before and the operation wasn't dangerous. The physicians agreed, the patient was ready to have anything done that offered to relieve his misery. While the physicians watched, Ambroise opened the prominent, strongly pulsating artery. The blood spurted and he allowed "two or more palettes," about six ounces, to flow before he controlled the bleeding. He intimated that he put a stitch through the skin and ligated the vessel, allowing the suture to remain several days before removing it. The pain ceased immediately and did not return. Ambroise said that the Prince gave him "an honorable present." In the 20th century, surgeons would revive this therapy for unilateral headache, this time considering it necessary to interrupt the sympathetic nerve fibers accompanying the artery.

Since Paré's day, this little village on the Gulf of Gascony has become the world-famous pleasure resort of Biarritz. He found it in the midst of a whaling season and, having read a book by Rondelet about whales, was interested in observing the methods the natives used to take them. He discussed this in his book on *Monsters and Prodigies* (Malgaigne, III, p. 779). Behind the village was a hill with a watch tower where the people kept a look out for the beasts' coming, which was signalled by the noise they made and the spray they blew when surfacing. When the watchman rang a bell, all the people ran to the boats drawn up on the shore, everything prepared for the hunt. They had many boats and small ships, with some men detailed for the single purpose of rescuing whalers who fell overboard. On each boat were ten skilled oarsmen and others who threw the harpoons, each identified with the owner's mark. Paré watched them drive their harpoons home, then sit back and ride their boats, towed by the animals in their frenzied dash for freedom, until they were exhausted. Then the men took the oars and dragged their captive to the beach, where they cut it up and divided it among the participants. Paré said that the meat had little value, but the tongue was dainty and was salted down for future use. The lard was kept to be eaten with peas during Lent. The fat also was used for fuel and to grease the boats. The whalebone was used to build fences, to make stays for ladies dresses, knife handles and other things. The vertebrae were used for stools and chairs. Ambroise sent one of these home to Paris to add to his museum.

The King made an excursion to Biarritz to see the whaling on 11 July. The next day he sailed for Bidache and the Court started on its return journey by land. Several men and horses died of sunstroke. They went by Dax, Tartas and back through Mont-de-Marsan. On 23 July, at Cazaire, it became so hot that the leaders changed the route of travel, going by night and sleeping by day. They penetrated the frankly Huguenot territory of Guyenne, where the attitude of the populace toward them took a decidedly cooler turn.

They found Angoulême still disordered by recent fights.

The Cathedral had been wrecked and the King furiously ordered the desecrators apprehended and executed. In a private Council meeting, however, Catherine was informed firmly that the laws against the Huguenots must be changed or she would have civil war on her hands. The tour turned westward toward La Rochelle, passing through Jarnac, Marennes, Brouage and St. Jean d'Angely, where Dr. Chapelain and Castellan were to die four years later.

On 14 September, 1565, the Court made a Grand Entry into La Rochelle, the acknowledged Huguenot capital. Although they were greeted by a great parade, in contrast to other such entries, no cannon salutes from the walls announced their approach. The Constable and his troops had entered the city the day before and had disarmed the place. The necessity of the precaution was not lost upon the young King. He exiled the Lieutenant-Governor, the Huguenot minister and six of the most prominent citizens. The cry of persecution rang in their ears as the Court left the city. The local power of the Huguenots irritated the King greatly and a sense of apprehension oppressed the party as they progressed across Angoumois, Aunis and Poitou. Gradually, they began avoiding the principal towns, going from château to abbey by side roads.

On 9 October, the party dined at Beaupréau, where the Prince de la Roche-sur-Yon became very sick and died the next day. Ambroise did not record the passing of his old friend, which occurred some three months after he had ligated the Prince's temporal artery. Presumably he was under the care of his physicians. The King did not want to eat in the house where the Prince had died, so he had dinner in the pretty park and slept in the abbey. The next day they went on to Le Loroux-Bottereau, a château between Anjou and Brittany.

On 11 October, the party reached the Loire at Chebiette. Finding the bridge destroyed, they crossed the river in barges to reach Nantes and entered the château from the river. On the following day, the Court formally entered the city through a specially built theatre, but the populace was so openly rebellious that the King remained practically confined to the guarded château, where he rested for three days. On 15 and 16 October, the entourage covered ten leagues to reach the Constable's town of Châteaubriant. In this comfortable environment, the party rested and relaxed for three weeks. Word reached them there that the Turks had been forced to lift the siege of Malta; the King ordered a huge bonfire lit in celebration.

From Châteaubriant the party took an oblique course to the Loire, running the gauntlet of both Catholic and Huguenot Councils, pleading, threatening and criticizing the conduct of the government. Advised against entering Saumur, the disillusioned Court went by Bauge to Bourgueil, thence to Langeais, where they entered friendly territory. They crossed the Loire and entered the King's own château at Plessis-les-Tours, where they stayed for ten days.

On a prolonged visit in such a place, it was common for the King, Catherine, or both, to take small groups to visit neighboring points of interest. These excursions were mentioned in Jouan's diary. While he made no note of a side trip to Orléans, there is a tradition (d'Eschevannes, p. 118) that it was during the course of this tour that the King visited Orléans and fell in love with Marie Touchet.[95] She was a beautiful and talented girl of fifteen, and the sixteen-year-old Charles met her while staying in the home of her father, Jean, who was a member of the King's Council. The Court was amused and delighted at the romance, but for the young lovers it was no passing fancy. When the Court moved on, Marie went too, and she remained the King's mistress as long as he lived.

While the Court was at Orléans, the wife of the Queen's coachman was brought to see Drs. Chapelain, Castellan and Paré (Malgaigne, III, p. 212; Hamby, p. 125). She had such pain in her right arm that she wanted to throw herself from the windows. A guard kept constant watch over her. The physicians were reminded of the case of the Lady of Bordeaux, and they decided to treat this patient similarly. Paré applied the potential cautery and after an opening was made, the pain ceased.

In contrast to the actual cautery, this potential cautery was a tissue-corroding agent used quite frequently in those days. In 1579, Paré recounted how he had learned of the preparation of such an agent (Malgaigne, III, p. 582; Hamby, p. 150). He put a piece of it the size of a pea on the arm of one of his servants to test its effect. "I swear to God," he wrote, "that in half an hour it had made an opening that would admit a finger, down to the bone, leaving a soft, moist scar." Ambroise begged the chemist to tell him how it was made, but that practical salesman refused him flatly. The more Paré entreated, the firmer became his refusal. Finally, Ambroise offered him enough velvet to make a pair of breeches. The chemist could refuse no longer. He let Paré have the secret of its manufacture on the condition that he would never give it to anyone else or write of it in his books. He complained that Paré gave away too many such secrets and was too liberal in communicating his knowledge. Paré promptly broke his promise and described its preparation in detail "for the benefit of all surgeons, not only in Paris, but in all the world." He called it the "velvet cautery," not only for the painless smoothness with which it worked and the soft scar it left, but also as a token of the price it had cost him. Ambroise then apparently felt that he needed to explain the violation of his promise, as he had done in the case of the puppy-oil secret he had learned in Turin. He said that when the chemist had sold him the secret, it was his no longer. Moreover, Paré did not feel that he had wronged the chemist; on the contrary, together they had rendered a valuable public service.

It was at this time too, probably, that Ambroise visited Paris with other members of the Court. They found the city in the midst of a grave epidemic of smallpox. Some of the courtiers contracted the disease and brought the infection back to the other members of the Tour.

In August of 1565, as was the custom, the King had given Ambroise the estate of Jean Gaultier, a foreign teacher in the medical school, who had died in the city (Le Paulmier, p. 199). Claude Gaultier, brother and heir of the deceased, living at Charpentras, entered a protest and petition to the King's Treasurer, asking that he be permitted to have his brother's estate. On 16 October, the court decided against him. Ten days later, while on a visit to the city, Paré went to his lawyers, de Netz and le Camus, at the Châtelet and made a voluntary bequest of the teacher's estate to his brother Claude. The reason given in the legal papers (Le Paulmier, p. 204) was that Claude was an old man of sixty years or more; he was poor and had to bring up four children. This example shows that Paré's generosity was not confined to his family and personal friends; he had a sense of justice far in advance of his time.

On Sunday, 1 December 1565, the Court took up its tour again, to Chenonceaux, to Blois, with short visits at each, and then started for Moulins, where a Grand Assembly of Notables had been called. The way led through Chevernay, Romorantin, Vierzon, Bourges, St. Just, Dun-sur-Auron, St. Menoux, and thus they approached Moulins. They entered the city on Sunday 22 December, and the King established his Court, celebrated Christmas and settled down for three months to transact important business.

While the Court was at Moulins, Paré was called with M. le Fèvre and Jacques Le Roy,[96] King's Physicians-in-Ordinary, to treat Madame de Castelpers' cook (Malgaigne, III, p. 320; Hamby, p. 130). While picking hops to make a salad, he was struck on the hand by an adder. He sucked out the venom and his tongue promptly swelled so greatly that he could hardly speak. The arm swelled "like a souffle," said Ambroise. The pain was extreme; the man fainted twice while being examined. The attendants washed out the man's mouth with brandy containing theriac and Paré incised the arm in several places to drain it. The cook was put into a warm bed to sweat and the next day was on his way to recovery.

In the midst of the important negotiations of the Assembly, the King developed an attack of smallpox, as did his sister Marguerite. During the illness, the King was bled by Antoine Portail (Malgaigne, II, p. 115; Hamby, p. 54), on the orders of Drs. Chapelain and Castellan. On opening the vein, the knife pricked the median nerve. The King cried out in pain. Paré immediately ordered the tourniquet loosened to prevent swelling and applied a compress over the incision. The arm went into violent spasm and pain shot through its entire length. Ambroise applied compresses wet with oxycrate to the arm and bandaged it firmly from fingertips to shoulder. Then the physicians and surgeons retired in consultation on the proper management of the case. They covered the arm with a plaster and replaced the compressing bandages, and the pain ceased. The King continued unable to flex or extend the arm for three months, but finally, "thanks to God," was cured perfectly without being deprived of any function.

The King had improved sufficiently by 23 March that he was able to go by litter to attend a tournament to which he had been invited, in Auvergne. Ambroise and the medical attendants accompanied him, going by way of St. Germain-des-Fosses and Vichy to Clermont, now called Clermont-Ferrand. Catherine's mother, Madelaine de la Tour d'Auvergne, had lived here, and Charles and the Queen visited her relatives.

While they were in Clermont, a Spanish Gentleman was presented to the King (Malgaigne, III, p. 341; Hamby, p. 133). As a gift of great value, he had brought the King a bezoar stone from Spain. This valued present was a concretion that is found in the stomach of various ruminants, but it was supposed to be an antidote against all poisons. The young King must have had an active mind and considerable curiosity; he called Paré in to ask him if indeed any drug protected against all poisons. Paré always tried to help the King reason things out for himself, instead of giving him categorical opinions. He explained that since venoms and poisons worked in various ways upon the body, it was unreasonable to expect any one agent to prevail against all of them.

When the Spanish Lord protested that the bezoar did indeed protect against all poisons, Paré suggested that the conflicting viewpoints could be resolved only by experimentation; if the King wished, the effect could be tried on a condemned criminal. The King immediately called the Provost of his house, M. de la Trosse, and asked if any criminal awaited the gallows. The Provost replied that a certain cook was to be hanged and strangled the next day for stealing two silver dishes from his master. The King explained that he wanted to test the bezoar against a definite poison. If the cook wanted to make the trial instead of being hanged, the King would pardon him if he survived. The cook agreed gladly, saying that he preferred poison in prison to hanging in public.

An apothecary then gave the cook a dose of a certain poison, followed immediately by a good dose of the bezoar. At once the cook began to vomit and to purge. He cried that his body was afire, and he drank large quantities of water. An hour later Paré requested M. de la Trosse to let him see the prisoner. He was sent into the dungeon with an escort of four archers. There he saw a pitiful sight. The poor cook was ambling about on all-fours like an animal, his tongue hanging out, his eyes and face flaming red; he was retching constantly, sweating profusely and bleeding from his mouth, nose, ears, anus and penis. Paré gave him a pint of oil to drink immediately, trying to help him. It was too late. The poor victim lived seven hours after taking the poison, crying that death on the gallows would have been much better.

Ambroise did an autopsy in the presence of M. de la Trosse and the four archers. The stomach was found corroded, black and dry. This indicated to Paré that the poison had been sublimate of mercury. The experiment having proved the worthlessness of the antidote, the King threw the bezoar into the fire. It burned.

Years later, after the death of the King, Paré was criticized severely by Dr. Gourmelen for having been the instigator of this "legal murder." This was an unusual charge; it was common practice for lesser noblemen than the King to make such human experiments on condemned criminals, even without their consent. It has been rumored that they sometimes were condemned for this specific purpose. Paré answered that it was more important for the King to be informed against such superstitions, and perhaps thereby avoid relying upon a false hope, than to have a criminal die in a manner somewhat different from the one to which he had been condemned originally. Lest one moralize too quickly in a vastly different environment, condemnation might better be directed against the justice that would hang a petty thief of two silver dishes. Paré's oft-demonstrated compassion insures that this experiment was not unusual in the times in which he lived.

On April 2, the Court left Clermont and started home, going via Riom, Ebreuil, Cosne, La Charité-sur-Loire and Entrain, to

Auxerre, which they reached on the 18th. Descending the Seine valley northward, they went to Sens, Nangis, Bray-sur-Seine, and then to Catherine's Château de Monceaux, near Meaux. Here they rested for a few days and on the first of May 1566, made a Grand Entry into Paris. The Tour had lasted two years, three months and eight days; covered forty-five hundred kilometers, and resulted in a disappointing failure. The passions of the country had not been cooled; in fact, the Conference of Bayonne had increased the suspicions and hostilities. The King had begun to understand the status of the country, but he had been torn between opposing factions and, being unable to dominate the situation, remained even more confused, frustrated and demoralized.

On his return to Paris, Paré became involved in a family tragedy. He never wrote of it, but the incident was seized upon gleefully by Gourmelen later in his attacks upon Paré's use of the ligature in amputations. For some unknown reason it became necessary for Gaspard Martin, barber-surgeon husband of Ambroise's older sister Catherine, to have his leg amputated. Paré did the operation in his usual manner, using the ligature for hemostasis, but unfortunately the patient died some days later. Cognizant of the mortality attending such operations at the time, modern surgeons would not be surprised at even Ambroise's loss of the patient, but Gourmelen attributed the result to the ligature alone.

CHAPTER IX

Civil War -- Trip to Flanders -- Surgical Writing
1566-1575

1567

E<small>ARLY IN</small> 1567, Paré engaged in a bit of unsuccessful professional politics. Traditionally, the King's Premier-Barber-Surgeon was the legal head, not only of the barber-surgeons but also of the surgeons of the Confraternity of St. Côme. This anomalous situation was supported by the Faculté de Médecine to preserve their own superiority over the surgeons (Le Paulmier, p. 66). After securing the sympathies and support of the King's Physicians, Paré petitioned the King to give his Premier-Surgeon, or a Board of his representatives, jurisdiction over all the practitioners of surgery in France. He proposed that two physicians should be associated with the Board, obviously a sop to the Faculté. On 7 May, 1567, the King sent the proposal to the Faculté for its advice. A committee of the Faculté consulted with all interested parties and both the Sworn-Surgeons and the Barber-Surgeons took alarm at the idea of a single effective authority over both groups. They joined with the Faculté then in recommending no change in the status quo. Paré's request was tabled. Not until the reign of Louis XIV were the surgeons finally freed from their subjection to the King's Premier-Barber-Surgeon.

ST. DENIS

Meanwhile, the uneasy religious truce faltered. Armed groups began gathering and finally the Royal Family itself had to make a night flight from its residence at Monceau to Paris to avoid capture by Condé's cavalry. Condé's troops then raced to take

Paris and on 10 November, 1567, clashed with the Royal army at St. Denis. The Catholics won, but at the cost of the seventy-five-year-old Constable Montmorency, whose spine was shattered by a pistol ball.

The wounded from St. Denis poured into Paris to be treated. Paré and his assistants were very busy. His most important patient was the Constable (Malgaigne, III, p. 733; Hamby, p. 190). At the request of Madame de Montmorency, the King sent Ambroise to treat him at his hotel, a portion of the park of which persists near the Porte d'Auteil. There Ambroise found the bold, seventy-five-year-old warrior who had fought, bravely always, and at times brilliantly, under five Kings of France, paralyzed below the waist. Sharing the fate of most patients so wounded before World War II, he rapidly developed bladder infection and uremia and died in coma within a few days. A suit of his chain-mail armor can be seen in the Metropolitan Museum in New York, hanging in a glass cage, for all the world resembling the pelt of a great bear. He may have been bigoted, single-minded, illiterate and, as has been charged by lesser men than himself, perhaps not overly bright, but he was a real fighting man of intense and constant loyalty, a knight who had outlived his era.

1568

While in Carcassone, in January of 1565, after the Court tour had passed through the plague-strickened Lyon area, Catherine and the King asked Paré to write a book on the causes, transmission and treatment of the plague. He had been working on it at odd moments since. Now the manuscript was ready. This was to be a less pretentious book than his last three, being designed as a work-book for busy surgeons, and perhaps even for young physicians. Ambroise chose as his publisher André Wechel, son of Christian Wechel, famous for his Latin and Greek editions (Doe, p. 56). André had succeeded his father in 1554, and was to have trouble because of suspected Huguenot sympathies, causing him to move to Frankfort the next year.

Paré's privilege for printing was granted on 4 May 1568, for nine years. The book, *Traicte De La Peste, De La Petite*

Verolle & Rougeolle: Avec Une brefue Description de la Lepre etc., contained two hundred seventy-five pages and no illustrations. He dedicated it to his friend Dr. Castellan. This was one of Paré's most systematic treatises; it ranks among the best of his writings, although it has little scientific value. At the end of the text appeared the motto: "Fin est la mort et principe de vie" (Death is the end and the beginning of life).

Malgaigne (Intro., p. cclxxii) implied that Paré had suffered his own attack of plague while on the Court Tour. This seems very unlikely, since he alluded to it only in passing (Malgaigne, III, p. 436; Hamby, p. 139), and as it had occurred long ago. Had it been so recent, he probably would have described the experience as vividly as he did his leg fracture of 1561.

The book lauded antimony as a drug of value in therapy, for which the Faculté castigated him. He did not reply, but left out the disputed passages when reprinting it in his *Oeuvres* in 1575, saying, "Some approve and strongly recommend antimony —. Since its use is disapproved by the gentlemen of the Faculté de Médecine, I shall proceed without writing of it here."

In a sort of an apology for Paré's writing on such a medical topic as the plague, Malgaigne (Intro., p. cclxxii) rather lamely excused him, but failed to stress the obvious reason. Paré himself stated positively that this was done on the direct order of the King and of the Queen-Mother.

About this time also, a book was published at Caen and at Paris by Julien Le Paulmier[97] entitled *Traicté de la nature et curation des playes de Pistole, Harquebouses et autres bastions à feu*, etc. (*Treatise on the Nature and Cure of Wounds by Pistol, Harquebus and Other Fire-Arms*, etc.) Le Paulmier was a Regent-Physician of the Faculté de Médecine of Paris, but he followed Paré's initiative in writing in French instead of Latin, perhaps in hopes of reaching the same readers. In his book, he blandly adopted and plagiarized Paré's arguments against the poisonous quality of gun-shot wounds and his method of controlling amputation hemorrhage with the ligature instead of the cautery. The plagiarism Paré might have overlooked, since he sincerely wanted these ideas accepted, but Le Paulmier attacked his method of dressing open wounds with large tents, and attributed to this method the high mortality rate among those wounded at Dreux, St. Denis and Rouen. This made Paré indignant. He began writing his rebuttal that appeared in his *Cinq Livres de Chirurgie,* to be published in 1572.

On 5 July, Paré lost an old and valued friend. Étienne de la Rivière died and was buried at St. Innocent's Church.

MONCONTOUR

Paré was with the King and the Court at Plessis-les-Toyrs, outside Tours, when news came of the victory for the Royal troops in a new battle at Moncontour. Almost simultaneously, the wounded started pouring into Tours. The King put Paré to work. Fortunately, he had plenty of help now. Pigray[98] and Portail were there, as was Guillaume du Bois and M. Siret, a surgeon of Tours. Du Bois was an old friend who had been a member of the College of Surgeons when Paré was admitted, and one of the Surgeons-in-Ordinary of the King, and of his father earlier. M. Siret was surgeon of the King's brother, the Duke d'Anjou, who was familiarly called Monseigneur. In his account of this engagement, Paré reported that the work was so heavy that neither physicians nor surgeons got any rest (Malgaigne, III, p. 725; Hamby, p. 183).

A Gentleman came to the Court then from the Count de Mansfeld,[99] Governor of Luxembourg and Knight of the Order of the King of Spain, with a plea to the King to send surgeons to dress him at Bourgueil (Malgaigne, III, p. 725; Hamby, p. 184).

Charles and his mother discussed the matter with Henri, the Marshal de Montmorency, son of the late Constable, who advised the King to send Paré to the Count. Charles at once said that someone else must go; he wanted Paré to remain with him. Montmorency pointed out that as the Count was a foreigner who had come as a volunteer to aid the Catholics at the command of the King of Spain, he was entitled to their best surgeon, especially since he had helped insure a victory. The King was persuaded then and agreed to let Ambroise go, on condition that he would return promptly. Ambroise was called and Charles ordered him to go find the Count where ever he might be, and to do everything possible to help him.

Paré rode to Bourgueil, a charming town forty-five kilometers west of Tours in the Loire valley. There he found his patient with his left elbow shattered by a pistol ball. Paré gave him letters from the King and the Queen-Mother and the Count was so pleased with Ambroise that he dismissed three or four other surgeons who had been attending him, including Nicole Lambert[100] and Richard Hubert. This didn't make Paré very happy, since he feared that the wound would be fatal. He found that many other Gentlemen had retreated to Bourgueil. They had followed Henri de Guise,[101] who had sustained a bad pistol wound of the leg, since they knew he would have good surgeons attending him. The Duke was reputed to be kind and generous and the wounded knew that he would help them all he could. Ambroise reported that the Duke indeed did furnish them with food, drink and other necessities, while he gave them the comfort of his art.

The Count de Ringrave, who had commanded a company of land squenets on the expedition that Paré had accompanied to Germany in 1552, was here also, injured by a pistol ball in the left shoulder. This was the same type of wound that had killed the King of Navarre and François de Guise, and Ringrave also died of it at the age of twenty-four (Malgaigne, III, p. 725; Hamby, p. 185).

Interestingly enough, M. Christophe de Bassompierre[102] had sustained an elbow wound like that of the Count de Mansfield. Christophe's father's sister was Mansfeld's wife. Paré treated both of these Gentlemen for three weeks, then took them back to Paris, where he operated upon Mansfeld's arm to remove carious bone fragments. The Count recovered "by the grace of God" and gave Paré "an honest reward, so I was as well pleased with him as he was with me, as he later demonstrated."

The Count de Mansfeld wrote to his friend, the Duke d'Ascot,[103] telling him how well Paré had treated his arm, that of Bassompierre and many others wounded at Moncontour. He suggested that the Duke request the King to send Paré to see and treat his wounded and failing brother, the Marquis d'Auret.[104] Since he told the story in considerable detail, and the detail better conveys the flavor of Paré's writing and thinking than can a summarization; it should be read from source (Malgaigne, III, p. 726; Hamby, p. 186). Most of the story is included in the several available reprints of Paré's *Apologie*.

The Duke d'Ascot sent a Gentleman to the King with a letter humbly begging him to do him the honor of sending Paré to see his brother, the Marquis d'Auret, who had been shot in the thigh about seven months earlier. The neighboring medical people had been unable to help him. The King sent for Paré and ordered him to go to M. d'Auret and to do all he could to cure him.

Conducted by two Gentlemen, Paré went to the Marquis at the Château d'Auret, a league and a half from Mons, in Heinault, now Belgium. He visited the Marquis as soon as he arrived, and told him that the King had ordered him to come and dress his wound. The Marquis was very happy to see him and expressed his gratitude to the King and to Paré.

Ambroise found the Marquis to have a high fever, his eyes sunken into a yellow, moribund face, his tongue dry and rough, his body emaciated and his voice low, "like a man very near death." He found his thigh swollen, purulent and ulcerated, draining green, fetid pus. On probing the wound, he found evidence of osteomyelitis extending from the knee almost to the groin. The leg was retracted nearly to the buttock, where there was a decubitus ulcer as large as the palm of the hand. The man was in constant pain, so he could neither sleep nor eat, although he could drink.

After examining the patient, Ambroise regretted his trip, since it appeared dubious that he could be cured. However, he resolved to do his best, and encouraged the Marquis that with the help of God, he would put him on his feet again. Paré then went to walk in the garden, where he prayed for God's help and planned his treatment. He was called to dinner then, and entering through the kitchen, he saw a huge cauldron where several kinds of meat and lots of good vegetables were boiling. He decided that the broth from this kettle was just what the Marquis needed for nourishment.

After dinner, all the physicians and surgeons who were in attendance assembled in conference in the presence of the Duke d'Ascot and several of his Gentlemen. Paré recounted the details of his examination and wondered why the leg had not been drained earlier. He was told that for almost two months they had been unable to even change the bed linen because of the pain the patient suffered. All the consultants gave their opinions of his condition; it was deplorable. Paré granted this, but insisted that since the Marquis was young, hope remained. He outlined his plan of treatment, and they agreed to it.

The consultation over, they went to the patient and Paré made three incisions into the thigh, draining a great deal of pus and removing several bone spicules. Two or three hours later a fresh bed was prepared and a strong man lifted him into it; the Marquis was very glad to be out of the dirty, stinking bed in which he had been for so long. Soon he asked to be left alone and he slept for several hours, much to the joy of his anxious relatives.

Later, the wounds were irrigated with Egyptiac[105] dissolved in either brandy or wine, were dressed with tents and were covered with a great plaster of diachalcitheos[106] dissolved in wine and were bandaged skillfully. The patient and his leg were massage, his hair was clipped and his head rubbed with soothing lotions. Sleep was encouraged by simulating the sound of rain by pouring water slowly from a height into a cauldron. He was given diluted wine to drink, since this lifted the spirits; his appetite improved and he began to eat better. Soon two of his surgeons and a physician were released, so only three remained with him.

Paré remained there for two months and saw many patients, rich and poor, who came from two or three leagues around for his attention. The Marquis had food and wine given these visitors, and cautioned Paré to see that this was done, to help them. Seeing the Marquis improve, Paré had a jester brought in to cheer him and musicians were hired to play for him. Within a month he was up in a chair and then was carried into the garden so he could visit with people who came from miles around to visit with him. He had them served wine and beer and they danced and sang for him in happiness over his recovery. Citizens came from Mons, and Gentlemen and Ladies from nearby châteaus visited him, for "he was greatly loved by the nobility and the common people, as much for his liberality as for his honesty and handsomeness, having a pleasant face and gracious speech, so that all who saw him were constrained to love him."

The chiefs of the city of Mons came on a Saturday and, as a token of affection for the Marquis, invited Paré to attend a dinner they would give in his honor. Ambroise was reluctant to go, thinking it out of place for him, a commoner, to accept such an invitation. The Marquis urged him to do it, since it actually was an expression of regard for himself. Paré reluctantly consented to go, assuring the Marquis that the hospitality of the citizens of Mons meant infinitely less to him than did the Marquis' own.

The next day, two coaches came to the château and Ambroise was taken to Mons. There he found a dinner ready, with the Chiefs of the city and their wives waiting to welcome him. They put him at the head of the table and they drank toasts to the health of the Marquis and to the man who had made it possible. After much celebrating, Ambroise was taken back to the château. Here the Marquis awaited him, eager to hear of his party. Ambroise made him very happy with his account of how he had received the honors as an agent for the Marquis.

The Marquis continued to improve, to get fat and to assume a healthy color. He got up on crutches and the wanted to pay a visit to his brother, the Duke d'Ascot, at his château at Beaumont. He traveled by litter, borne by relays of eight men. At each village, the occupants gathered to meet him, and urged his party to drink with them. Paré said that it was only beer, but he believed that had it been wine or Hippocras, they would have served it as willingly. The local men then argued over who should have the honor of helping carry the litter to the next village.

When they arrived at the château, they found more than fifty Gentlemen invited by the Duke awaiting them. They offered prayers of gratitude for the Marquis' recovery and held open-house, making merry for three days. At dinner, Paré was "always at the upper end of the table" and everyone "drank carouses" to him and the Marquis. Ambroise said that they tried to get him drunk, but they couldn't, for he only drank as he was accustomed to. After dinner, the Gentlemen fenced, tilted at the ring and disported themselves as at a holiday.

A few days later they departed and in farewell, the Duchesse d'Ascot took a diamond "worth well over fifty crowns" from her finger and gave it to Ambroise in gratitude for his help to her brother-in-law. At home the Marquis began to walk alone on the garden on crutches. Ambroise began to ask permission to depart, since he was needed no longer, but the Marquis was reluctant to let him go. To accustom him to his absence, Paré requested permission to visit Antwerp. To this the Marquis gladly assented and sent his Maitre-de'Hôtel and two pages to take care of him. They went by way of Malignes and Brussels and there and at Antwerp the Chiefs of the cities gave dinners in his honor, happy over the recovery of the Marquis. After two and a half days at Antwerp they returned to the Marquis, whom Paré regaled with accounts of the esteem and affection these people had for him, the Marquis.

Finally, after another week, the Marquis reluctantly let him go. He gave Ambroise "a present of great value and had him accompanied to the door of his house in Paris by the Maitre-d'Hôtel and two pages. Paré ended the account with the sad note that the Spaniards had since ruined and demolished the Château d'Auret and had sacked, pillaged and burned all the villages belonging to the Marquis, because he would not join their evil party in the ruin of the Low Countries.

This little story gives us tremendous insight into the intimate character of Ambroise Paré as he entered his sixtieth year. His hopes and fears are honestly exposed. His humble supplication of Divine assistance in his problems is testimony of the persistence of his faith through a tumultous lifetime of practice in a period when surgery was a dangerous and bloody business. Justly deserved honors did not upset his sense of proportion; he remained "humble" even at the head of the tables of the mighty. There might be another lesson here for surgeons too. Despite his primitive and now antiquated notions of pathology, extending to him from Hippocrates and Galen, his painstaking utilization of details of empirical care acquired from his own controlled experience let him succeed in the treatment of complicated cases that might well tax the skill of the modern surgeon, despite all his scientific resources.

This trip marked another turning point in Paré's life; it was his last army expedition. He had established his reputation and became famous as a result of his compassion for the poor, ignorant, wounded soldier. That this led directly to his solicitation by the mighty, even five Kings, apparently impressed him only slightly; the lessons he wrote in his books were intended primarily for the young surgeon, treating the common soldier. King Henri II, François de Guise, the Constable Montmorency, the King de Navarre, the Prince de Condé—all were gone. A newer breed ran the show. Ambroise was sixty years old now, and twenty more would remain to him, in which he would consolidate, polish and disseminate his knowledge within the profession. He would treat the patients who flocked to his shop and follow them to their homes whenever necessary; for this he would be richly rewarded, but this was the end of an era for him.

1570

Ambroise continued to add to his museum of curiosities, and this year received a skeleton of a twin fetus having a single head. The monster had been delivered in Tours the year before by René Ciret, a Master Barber-surgeon "whose renown was famous through the whole country of Tourraine," as Paré said, adding, "if it were not, I would give him added praise" (Malgaigne, III, p. 9; Hamby, p. 109).

Political affairs continued hectic. Charles IX was married on 26 November 1570 to the Archduchesse Elizabeth, daughter of the Emperor Maximillian II[107] of Austria. She was a charming woman whom the French took to their hearts immediately. Marie Touchet calmly retained her place as the King's mistress.

Amidst all the distractions of the Court and of his busy practice, Paré was hard at work writing. He was finishing his *Cinq Livres de Chirurgie, Five Books of Surgery,* for which he had obtained the Royal Privilege two years earlier. This book contained instructions on bandaging, on fractures and dislocations, on bites and stings of venomous animals and insects and on gout. It also contained his *Apologie touchant les playes faites par harquebuses*, responding to Julien Le Paulmier's attack upon his method of treating wounds, which had appeared a year earlier. He was also working on another, *Deux Livres de Chirurgie, Two Books of Surgery*, containing his ideas on human reproduction, the development of the fetus and delivery, an account of monsters, both actual and mythological, and on wounds of the nerves and on dentistry.

Both of these books contained largely new material and included much evidence of research and of reporting of ideas of both ancient and modern writers on the subjects. The *Five Books* had forty-one wood-cuts, some used and some new. The *Two Books* had eighty-seven, many of them new. These were being cut for printing. His printer, André Wechel was back in Paris after a period of exile, preparing to publish his books.

1572

Sometime in the spring of 1572, Wechel finished printing Paré's *Cinq Livres de Chirurgie*. This book also was written for the young surgeon and, as he had done before, Paré promised to write more if this one were well received. It was dedicated "To the Very Powerful and Very Christian King of France, Charles, Ninth of the Name, by Ambroise Paré, His first surgeon and very humble servant." It had four hundred seventy pages, with forty-one illustrations, as mentioned earlier, and Paré's wood-cut portrait. This portrait was reproduced from the 1561 book on Head Injuries, the age note altered from forty-five to fifty-five. There were eight wood-cuts of chemical apparatus, more of which had been planned, but Paré stopped at this point after learning that a colleague, Phillippe de Beauregard was writing an illustrated book on distillations. Doe (p. 71) was unable to find this book.

Doe commented also on the date of appearance of the *Five Books*. Paré's reply to Le Paulmier first appeared here, in the book on luxations. Not wanting to respond directly to Paré's reply, Le Paulmier had a vituperous attack upon him published by a barber-surgeon, *Discours des harquebusades en forme d'epistre pour respondre a certaine apologie publiee par Ambroise Paré*, p. J. M., Compagnon-Barbier, Lyons, 1572. This appeared on 20 March 1572, meaning that Paré's *Five Books of Surgery* was distributed some time earlier.

Within a few months, although it was dated 1573, Wechel also released Paré's *Deux Livres de Chirurgie*. Doe noted that the book must have appeared before 24 August, the date of the Massacre of St. Bartholomew. Having already been driven temporarily from Paris for his Huguenot involvement, Wechel was marked as a victim of the massacre and was not killed only because Hubert Languet, agent of the Elector of Saxony, was living in his house. As soon as possible thereafter, Wechel emigrated permanently and set up his press in Frankfort. He was not in Paris in 1573.

This book was written as the result of a conversation with the Duke d'Uzés, who had urged Paré to put into print what he had told him about the formation and development of the fetus. Paré added other information as mentioned earlier and dedicated it to the Duke. This volume contained six hundred nineteen pages, with eighty-seven wood-cut illustrations and a slightly altered reprint of the portrait from the *Five Books*. These two volumes on surgery contained almost eleven hundred pages of text, a monumental task of preparation. At the end of the last book Paré announced that he was planning to publish all of his books in one volume, adding new material.

THE ST. BARTHOLOMEW'S DAY MASSACRE

While Ambroise was preoccupied with his publications, tragedy was stalking his country. The Catholics had become convinced that the growing menace of the Huguenot cause had to be eliminated. On 18 August, the Princess Marguerite de Valois was married to Henri, King de Navarre, and the Huguenot leaders were all in Paris, either by desire or by Royal command.

On Friday, 22 August, 1572, the Admiral Coligny was walking in the rue des Fosses-St. Germain-l'Auxerrois, just east of the Louvre, returning from the Louvre to his home, reading a letter.

A shot smashed two fingers of his right hand and lodged in his left arm. He wheeled and pointed out the house from which the shot had come, in the cloister of St. Germain-l'Auxerrois, belonging to a man named Maureval, a tutor of Henri de Guise. The Admiral walked home to the Hôtel de St. Pierre, in rue Bethisy, and sent word of the attack to the King and Catherine. Catherine sent Paré to treat Coligny.

Ambroise amputated the two smashed fingers, opened the wounded left arm and dressed the wounds. At two o'clock in the afternoon the King, Catherine and a party of Royalists visited him. They departed later, the King very upset over the attack upon the Admiral, whom he loved greatly. In several conferences during the night, the Royal party came to the conclusion that the Admiral was subverting the King and that he must die. The conferences continued intermittently, tremendous pressure being put upon the King to agree to the assassination. War with the Huguenots seemed inevitable, and it would give the Royal party a tremendous advantage if their leaders, in their hands in Paris, were exterminated. At last they wore the King down and he yielded, saying "—I consent, but see to it that not only he, but all the Huguenots in Paris die, so that none remains to reproach me!"

The accounts of the horror that followed are confused and contradictory. At any event, the Catholic party was ready. Henri de Guise led his troops to the Admiral's Hotel; an entrance was forced and Coligny was murdered. His body was thrown through a window into the court-yard where Guise identified it and rode away. The bells of St. Germain-l'Auxerrois began tolling and the Catholics poured into the streets bent upon exterminating the Huguenots before they could arrange to protect themselves. The Huguenots fought back blindly or with preplanned efficiency, depending upon their foresightedness. As in all such conflicts, many entirely innocent of any serious attachment to either side went down and more died at the hands of the criminal elements suddenly given the opportunity to turn a profitable bit of murder unnoticed. Paré is said to have escaped over the roof-tops from Coligny's house and he returned to the Louvre where the King kept him in his own bedroom all night for his protection.

St. Bartholomew's Day, Sunday, 24 August, was a day of carnage in which thousands died in the city streets and in their invaded homes. Henri de Navarre and Henri de Condé were saved by the King's order also and were kept in the Louvre for their protection. The rage then spread to the provinces and murder walked the land. In many towns under either Catholic or Huguenot control, the chiefs took over with firm hands and no overt acts of violence were tolerated.

Several Court physicians and surgeons identified as Huguenots also survived the massacre. Simon Pietre[108] and Jean Riolan took refuge in the Abbaye St. Victoire and Jean Mazille, Charles' Premier-Physician, remained at the Court until the King's death.

Despite this severe blow at their leadership, the Huguenots struck back and in November the Fourth War of Religion was on. La Rochelle was their capital, and in February 1573 siege was laid to the town. It dragged along until July, when Charles signed a peace with them. Concessions made to the Huguenots were greater than they had ever enjoyed and the total effect was to nullify the blood-letting of St. Bartholomew's Day.

Never a strong personality, the King began to undergo a decided chance in character. Obsessed by a strong sense of guilt over the massacre that he now began to see had accomplished nothing basic, he suffered such remorse that he slept poorly, beset by nightmares dripping with blood. He drove himself physically, riding twelve or more hours a day at the hunt and spending other long hours at hard physical exercise at tennis and at a forge where he worked on horse-shoes, cannon-founding and other blacksmithery. He probably thus prepared the ground for his fatal attack of tuberculosis the following year.

This must have been an unhappy year at the Court for Ambroise also. Charles was a good friend of his, and he had practically helped to raise the boy to manhood. He was intensely patriotic and must have suffered at the sight and the knowledge of what was happening to the King and to his country in the name of religion. Apparently, his private life was a happy one in general, barring the sorrow over the deaths of his two children, but this also was a commonplace at the time. Jeanne Mazelin must have been a good wife, to have so managed his household that he was able to accomplish the things he did. Now, on Wednesday, 4 November, 1573, she died at the age of fifty-three, leaving Ambroise in charge of his thirteen year old daughter Catherine and his nineteen year old orphaned niece Jeanne. She was buried on the same day at St. André-des-Arts. It is only from church and court records, discovered by Le Paulmier, that these details are known; no personal memoirs have come down to us from Ambroise himself, even Malgaigne knew nothing of them.

Beyond his own personal sorrow, the loss of his efficient partner must have faced Ambroise with great problems. He had a tremendous practice requiring several apprentices and assistants, some of whom lived with him in his house and required personal supervision. His Court duties kept him away from home a great deal of the time and he never knew when he might be sent or taken out of Paris for periods of days or weeks. The unrest of the city laid grave responsibilities on householders to maintain their own personal safety, as well as to procure supplies necessary for daily living. Certainly the responsibilities were too great for him to consider leaving on the shoulders of two teen-aged girls, with all the assistance possible from surrounding relatives. Under these circumstances, one may well view sympathetically what might otherwise be considered the unseemly haste with which he found himself a new wife.

No record of the circumstances leading to the bethrothal has been found, but Le Paulmier (p. 209) reprinted the notary's record of the marriage contract signed between Paré and Jacquelin Rousselet on 31 December 1573. In the party of witnesses were her father, Jacques Rousselet, ordinary Equerry of the King's stables, her mother Mary Boullaie and twenty-six "privileged bourgeois of Paris." Ambroise Paré, Premier-Surgeon and Councillor of the King had as his witness his friend and neighbor Hilaire de Briou, Master-Apothecary and grocer. Jacquelin's parents pledged for her dowry five thousand gold livres to be paid the day before the wedding. Paré pledged five hundred gold livres a year, secured by rents from his property and the lifetime use of the Maison de la Vache, for which she would get two hundred livres annually. In the case children survived him, the dowry would be reduced to three hundred livres a year. In case of the death of Ambroise, Jacquelin would get her clothes, luggage and jewelry to the value of five hundred livres. In case of her death, Ambroise would retain his clothes, arms, horses and surgical instruments to a similar value. As signing witness, Jacquelin had Robert Boullaie, her first cousin, Secretary to the First President of Dauphine, M. François Bouteroue, Advocat in the Court of the Parlement. Paré's witness was M. de Briou. We don't know Jacquelin's age, but she survived Ambroise by sixteen years, dying in 1606.

1574

On Sunday 3 January, 1574, the marriage bans were published in St. Severin, Jacquelin's parish church. Although Paré's old church, St. André-des-Arts, has been razed, St. Severin remains in the block between the rue St. Jacques and the rue-des-Prêtres-St. Severin, two blocks from the left bank of the river. A part of the facade persists from the 13th century. To the right is the old cemetery ground enclosed behind and on the south side by the low arcade and the cells of the cloister.

Tradition has it that this cemetery was the site of the first recorded operation for removing a bladder stone in January of 1474, just a hundred years before Paré's wedding there. Desiring to find a way of handling such problems, physicians asked permission of King Louis XI to have the operation performed experimentally upon an archer of Meudon, who had such a stone, and who also was in prison, condemned to be hanged for robbery and sacrilege. He had burglarized the church of Meudon. The operation was believed done successfully upon the archer by Germain Collot, the patient recovering and going free, both of his stone and of the rope. Alas for such romances, however; in his tenacious manner Malgaigne (Intro., cliv) tracked the story down. There is no evidence that a surgeon or even an "inciseur" named Germain Collot ever lived in Paris. The story had been recorded by a registrar of the Hôtel-de-Ville named Jean de Troyes in the *Chronique scandaleuse*, but the description is that of an entirely different type of operation, involving opening the peritoneal cavity.

On Saturday, 9 January, Ambroise went to the Châtelet and there before his lawyers (Le Paulmier, p. 217) made an irrevocable donation to his niece, Jeanne Paré, of a house on his property (house E on the plan in Le Paulmier, p. 172). It was surrounded on two sides by the Paré courtyards and had access to the Place St. Michel via an alley running between the houses of M. de Pichonnat and of Méry de Prime. Its value was estimated at one thousand gold livres. In addition he willed her an annual sum of one hundred livres to come from rents on his property. Ambroise reserved the use of the house and the rents during his lifetime. If Jeanne died childless, these were to revert to his estate. In the midst of all his distractions, Ambroise was thoughtful of the future of his dependents.

On the following Wednesday, 13 January, Paré returned to the lawyers (Le Paulmier, p. 212) with the contracting parties and declared himself satisfied with two thousand livres of dowry instead of the original five thousand. This was paid him on 30 January, instead of the 17th as the contract had specified. Apparently, the Rousselets had a little trouble raising the sum within the legal time limit. The wedding was performed on 18 January 1574 in Jacquelin's church, St. Severin.

During the spring the overworked body of the frail and distraught King began to break down. Paré's old adversary, Dr. Julien Le Paulmier, was getting nowhere treating the young man's intractable insomnia. Dr. Mazille was disturbed by the exhaustion and finally the lung hemorrhages that followed the King's exertions. Paré is said to have remarked that this was aggravated by the King's habit of prolonged horn-blowing while riding at the hunt, at which he persisted feverishly. Finally he was forced to bed and, on the edge of collapse, was taken from St. Germain-en-Laye to Paris, where he went to the house of M. de Retz. Soon afterwards he was moved to Vincennes; he refused to return to the Louvre, the scene of his most unhappy memories. At Vincennes he was bedridden for almost three months, sweating and coughing blood. On Thursday, 26 May, a formal consultation was held by his physicians, who held no hope for him. Charles ordered a Regency to handle his affairs and appointed his mother. He swore his Captains to support his brother Henri, now King of Poland, and summoned Henri de Navarre for a conference.

On Sunday, 30 May, 1574, the twenty-three-year-old King Charles IX died in the thirteenth year of his reign. At four o'clock on the next day, Paré performed the autopsy and embalmed the body. Professional witnesses of the autopsy included the late King's Premier-Physician, Dr. Jean Mazille and Physicians-in-Ordinary Michel Vaterre,[109] Alexis Gaudin,[110] Regnault Vigor,[111] Pierre le Fèvre, M. de St. Pont,[112] Simon Piètre, François Brigard,[113] Pierre Lafille,[114] and Loys Duret.[115] Surgeons mentioned by Le Paulmier included Jean d'Amboise,[116] Guillaume de Bois, Antoine Portail, M. Eustace, Jacques Dionneau, Nicole Lambert, Jean Cointeret and Jacques Guillemeau (Le Paulmier, p. 84). Many of these people were old friends and acquaintances of Ambroise; he mentioned some of them repeatedly in his case reports. It is interesting that Paré never published the findings of this autopsy. He had described the autopsy findings in the case of King Henri II (Malgaigne, II, p. 25; Hamby, p. 26) and the details of Charles' nerve injury by Portail; perhaps nothing unusual was found in the autopsy of a young man dead of pulmonary tuberculosis, even though a King.

Henri, Duke d'Anjou was in Cracow, where he had been crowned King of Poland on 9 May, 1573. He became King Henri III of France on the death of Charles. Encouraged by his past energy and generalship in the Religious Wars during the lifetime of Charles IX, France had looked forward eagerly to having in him a true King who would unite the county. On his return a strange revulsion set in; he seemed to have undergone a complete change of character. No longer war-like, he no longer rode a horse; he secluded himself from the people and spent his time in the company of a group of young fops and queer young men with whom he had surrounded himself in Poland. The affairs of the country he left to his mother and the politicians, in a period when a fresh, vigorous hand on the reins was sorely needed.

As he had served his father and his two brothers before him, Paré continued to serve this strange young King, Henri III. He was reappointed Premier-Surgeon and Councellor. He also continued his busy practice and writing up the findings of his autopsies. On 27 July, he did an autopsy on Madame Roger. He found the uterus to be enlarged and, not wanting to dissect it alone, took it home to dissect the next day. He listed seventeen people who came to his house to witness it; they included the cream of the profession in Paris, physicians as well as surgeons and barber-surgeons (Malgaigne, III, p. 724; Hamby, p. 101).

On 30 November, Paré obtained the King's Privilege, signed at Avignon, for nine years to publish a book of his collected works. Since about 1570, he had been planning to publish a complete treatise on surgery, including all its ancillary fields from human conception to autopsy, even including the proper manner of making out reports of findings. His last two works, the *Five Books* and the *Two Books of Surgery* had been written with that specific purpose in mind. Paré must have been working on this collection, altering and rewriting his material for some time; it must have been in fairly polished form by now. Some time before this, Paré and his old friend and pupil Portail must have had a serious misunderstanding. As Malgaigne noted (III, p. 328; Hamby, p. 82), when describing his own leg fracture in 1564, Paré mentioned Portail as one of his attendants. In getting his complete works together now for publication, he dropped Portail's name from the list and never mentioned him again except very casually.

André Wechel had fled Paris after St. Bartholomew's Day, so Paré needed another publisher. He chose Gabriel Buon, a successful publisher who, with two associated publishers, had issued the first French version of the Bible in 1566. He was to issue all successive French editions of the *Oeuvres* during Paré's lifetime. After Buon's death in 1597, his widow, Jeanne Rondel, carried on the business and issued the fifth edition in 1598. After her death, their son Nicholas would print the rest of the Paris editions through 1628 (Doe, p. 107).

1575

On 6 January, 1575, Paré, Jacques Guillemeau and Antoine de

Bieux, a Master barber-surgeon of the Faubourgs St. Germain-des-Prés, met in consultation (Malgaigne, II, p. 745; Hamby, p. 104). The patient was a previously healthy and happy young woman of twenty-five or thirty years. She had had no children by her first marriage, but after the second, four years earlier, developed signs suggesting pregnancy. Gradually, a sense of disagreeable perineal pressure developed, then retention of urine, and pain became unbearable. She was examined by Christophle Mombeau, a neighborhood barber-surgeon friend. He told Paré that, finding the perineun swollen, he had done the usual things, applying poultices and plasters that stopped the pain. Then between the labia appeared a mass that drained vari-colored pus. The sense of pressure returned; for two years she felt as if a lead ball shifted in her pelvis when she turned in bed. To void or go to stool she had to shift this weight with her hands. When she walked she felt that something between her legs blocked their motion. She developed intermittent, generalized complications suggesting infection. Harassed and impatient, she finally heeded the advice of a woman quack and took antimony ten days before Paré saw her. This purged her violently and something prolapsed. For nine days she had had no more bowel movements and had not voided for four days. Friends advised her to call in the surgeons.

They found a blackened, purulent mass protruding from the vulva and decided that it must be removed. On alternate days they made gentle, painless traction on the mass, which finally came away. Paré did not indicate whether or not this required any other outside assistance. The tumor was examined by the surgeons, and by Drs. Alexis Gaudin, le Fèvre and de Violanes[117] and they concluded that it was the uterus. An ovary was attached to it, as well as a membrane they considered a hydatid mole which had become infected, ruptured and expelled.

The patient made a gratifying recovery and was well for three months. Then she developed pleurisy and a high fever, of which she died. The attendants performed an autopsy. They found no uterus, but in its place was a hard scar "Nature had made during the brief three months that remained, to try to replace what had been lost."

Ten years later, in his vicious attack upon Paré, Compérat (see p. 187) said the autopsy actually showed the uterus to be intact and named as witnesses M. de Baillif,[118] King's Physician in the Faculté de Médecine and Sworn-Surgeon Loys le Brun.[119] In his footnote following this case report, Malgaigne remarked that the facts were "impossible to judge at this late date," and wished that Paré had commented upon it in his later editions. Packard (p. 122) thought that while Paré and the other crude pathologists might have been mistaken about the identity of the uterus, it is impossible to believe that he had deliberately lied about it.

On 9 October, 1574, the Duchesse de Lorraine, Catherine's daughter Claude, delivered twin daughters in Nancy. She did not improve and the King sent Dr. Marc Miron[120] to her. Later Catherine sent her own Premier-Physician, Dr. Vigor, to help him. In January, 1575, the King sent Paré to Nancy to see his sister. Le Paulmier (p. 85) recorded the payment made by the Court for the trips; Paré got one hundred and twenty-five livres, a hundred less than was given Vigor for his journey; Vigor spent a month at least longer at the task, however. Paré rode horseback by post over the familiar road to Nancy. Despite the ministrations of the Royal attendants, the Lady continued to decline and died on 21 February 1575, at the age of twenty-eight.

While in Nancy, Paré renewed his acquaintance with the Duke's surgeon, Nicholas Picart, whom he had met on his visit there with the Court in 1564. Ambroise was impressed with an apparatus called an "ambi" which Picard had perfected for reducing shoulder dislocations. It was essentially a long wooden lever to which the arm was bound; it had a concavity at its end to fit into the axilla on the top side and another beneath to engage on an upright, such as the top of a chair-back or a more formal wooden column adjustable for height. By downward leverage on the arm, the short end forced the head of the humerus upward and allowed it to reenter its socket. A crude form of such an instrument had been described by Hippocrates, but Picart's version was an improvement. Paré described and illustrated Picart's invention and others, giving him full credit for them (Malgaigne, II, p. 377), thus preserving the memory of the Lorraine surgeon, whose name otherwise would have been forever lost. Paré's writings on luxations were complete at this time, so the notation did not appear in the first edition of his *Oeuvres,* but was reserved for the second, in 1579. Beyond mentioning her as the reason for his visit to Nancy, Paré gave no other account of the Duchesse's fatal illness. Probably his surgical services were not required.

After the fatal accident to her beloved Henri II, Catherine could not live in the Palace des Tournelles, and she commissioned the architect Philibert de L'Orme to build a new one for her, the Tuilerie Palace, west of the Louvre. Among the artists working on the new palace was the famous ceramist, Bernard Palissy.[121] During Lent, and Easter was on 3 April in, 1575, Palissy gave a series of three lectures to which Paré subscribed. Le Paulmier (p. 86) listed the group of subscribers.

CHAPTER X

Les Oeuvres d'Ambroise Paré The Final Years
1575-1590

On 22 April, 1575, the printing of Paré's *Oeuvres* was completed. Ambroise was on excellent terms with many members of the Faculté de Médecine as his references to them attest, but officially the body jealously guarded its prerogatives in the strictest sense and let no personal considerations intervene. On 5 May, officials of the Faculté demanded of the Parlement their right to pass upon the book prior to its sale. On 28 May, they invoked a decree of 1535 to the effect that books on medicine and surgery could not be published without their approval. They emphasized that Paré was an uneducated barber-surgeon who had been admitted inappropriately to the College of Surgery of St. Côme. They implied that the College should join them in their protest. According to Doe (p. 106), the matter was to have been considered on 31 May, but Paré had the case deferred to permit him to prepare his defense. On 9 July, before University deputies, Gourmelin, Dean of the Faculté, condemned the book as immoral and contrary to the best interests of the State. The Faculté demanded examination of the book by the Parlement before it was put on sale.

In response, Paré published a little quarto, fifteen-paged pamphlet entitled *Response de M. Ambroise Paré, Premier Chirurgien du Roy, aux calomnies d'aucuns Médicines et Chirurgiens, touchant ses oeuvres.* (*Response of Ambroise Paré, Premier Surgeon of the King, to the calumnies of certain physicians and surgeons, concerning his Works*). Le Paulmier (pp. 222-248) reprinted the entire memoir in its original form, since he knew of only one copy extant. Ambroise first addressed the court, informing them that the primary objection of the Faculté was to his publication in plain, understandable French, since they feared that such information broadcast would tend to make their services less necessary. Moreover, they feared that a better informed group of barber-surgeons would further encroach upon their practice. Being unwilling to attempt to justify these selfish attitudes, his detractors found it necessary to attack him on other lines. They raised moral issues, proclaiming parts of the book indecent and unfit for the eyes of the innocent.

Paré then proceeded methodically to his defense. He showed that Hippocrates and Galen had written in their own native languages and that the public had not suffered from such broad diffusion of information. He noted that his book on *Generation and Monsters* contained much that had been written by others and that his entire section was largely a reprint of his 1573 edition, which the Faculté had not found it necessary to censor. His descriptions of the anatomy of the genitalia, of pregnancy, abortion, sterility, hermaphroditism, etc., had included work previously published by others, to which his own observations had been added. He noted that "It is one thing to treat of the Civil Morality in moral philosophy for the instruction of tender young ladies and quite another to speak truly of matters natural to physicians and surgeons as I have done to teach men."

Against the accusation of false quotations, Ambroise went through the book, giving line and page of his sources, quoting authors verbatim. Where objection was raised concerning his opinion in disputed matters, he quoted authorities supporting his viewpoint. Where the truth of his reports of his surgical experiences was doubted, he listed physicians and surgeons who had witnessed them and could verify his statements. Objection had been made that his story of the fatal trial of the bezoar stone on the thief was unnecessarily brutal, defaming the name of the late King. Paré quoted a similar trial by Pope Clement VII of an oil supposed to be an antidote. He emphasized that the thief had freely elected to take the test, since he might go free, and preferred to die of poison in prison rather than by the rope.

He commented then that the test disabused the King of the value of the false antidote, and the thief would have died as certainly had he not made the trial. He pointed out that while he condemned magic as the work of devils, he had carefully excluded from this category the miracles of saints as being beyond his field of experience.

The Doctors had taken him to task for advocating the use of antimony in medical diseases. He replied that this drug would no more kill a person than would rhubarb or another drug, if given under proper conditions, and that virulent diseases require strong drugs, which might of themselves kill, whatever drug was used.

His detractors said that he had served only two kings. He reminded them that he had served the late King of Navarre, that Henri II had appointed him on the advice of the King of Navarre, that Charles IX had loved and esteemed him, and that Henri III had valued him enough to keep him in service as his Premier-Surgeon and had used his services on several occasions. Moreover, he had been sent to serve several great Lords whom he had treated and whom God had healed. Interestingly, he did not mention having served François II, although he was one of his official surgeons and had shared the condemnation of surgeons falsely accused of having poisoned him.

He concluded his defense: "On my part, I consider nothing in my book pernicious for being in our common tongue. So the divine Hippocrates had written in his language, which was known and understood by women and girls, speaking no other language. As for myself, I have written in French only to instruct the young surgeon, and not to have my book handled by idiots and mechanics."

The case was tried on 14 July. Finally, the court ordered that all parties to the action should deposit their pleas and arguments with the public ministry within three days. It confirmed the decree of 1535 and adjourned. As Le Paulmier (p. 93) reported, the decision of the trial court is not recorded. Apparently a settlement was made, for the book went on sale and was promptly sold out. The disputed passages were retained and were reprinted in the next edition. In that edition, only the book on Fevers was omitted as such, but its materials was included by dispersing it through other sections.

LES OEUVRES D'AMBROISE PARE

This book must have been a source of great satisfaction to Ambroise. Gabriel Buon did a fine job of publication and it was a credit to its author. The blocks from which its two hundred and ninety-five illustrations were printed were valued at a thousand écus and were given as a wedding present to Claude Viart[122] when he married Paré's niece Jeanne in 1577.

Paré's *Works* was a folio edition of nine hundred and forty-five pages of text and thirty-three leaves, with a classical title page depicting an elliptical plaque bearing the title: *Les Oeuvres de M. Ambroise Paré Counseiller, et Premier Chirurgien du Roy. Auec les figures & portraicts tant de l'Anatomie que des instruments de Chirurgie, & de plusiers Monstres. Le tout diuise en vingt six livres, comme il est contenu in la page suyuante.* (*The Works of Ambroise Paré, Councillor and Premier Surgeon of the King. With pictures and illustrations both of Anatomy and of Surgical Instruments, and of several Monsters. The whole divided into twenty-six books, as listed on the next page.*) On a lower half-circular plaque, curved side down, is the inscription: *A Paris, Chez Gabriel Buon. 1575. Auec Priuilege du Roy.*

These plaques were ornately mounted on an engraved support resembling a vertically elongated architectural rectangle having a flat cornice with a wide arc above it. In the center is a shield bearing three fleurs-des-lys, the whole surmounted by a crown with palm fronds. Seated on each side of the shield and facing it are half-draped, garlanded angels, each bearing a trumpet from which hangs a banner ornamented with a crowned capital H. On each side of the body of the title plaque are fluted columns, between which and the plaque are garlanded, classically-draped female figures supporting shields bearing coats of arms. The columns are supported on narrow rectangular bases roughly a third the height of the columns; the faces of the base blocks are decorated with the crowned device earlier used by Henri II, a capital H with intertwined crescents the tips of which join the extremities of the uprights of the H. These crescents were ostensibly meant during Henri's lifetime to represent C's, for Catherine. The combination of the C with its tips against the uprights of the H, of course, produced a D which, to the sophisticated, represented Diane de Poitiers, Henri's mistress. After Henri's death, Catherine had all the alterable devices changed by prolonging the tips of the Cs beyond the limits of the Hs, destroying the suggestion of the D, thus excluding Diane from this close association. Remnants of the original devices can still be seen unaltered where they were done in stone in high relief, as on the wall of the Louvre, at Chenonceaux and other places. In Paré's engraving, the edge of the H was distinctly so shaded that the suggestion of the D was evaded. So tedious can become the details of even the engraver's art in politics! Between the base of the title panel and the supports of the two lateral columns are nude infants depicted in mirror-image, one upraised arm grasping a descending band of drapery, the other resting on its elbow, the hand with pointing index finger crossing the figure's chest. The foot of the entire superstructure rests upon swirled conventions of foliage and fruits. The effect of the entire page is rich, dignified and in excellent, if somewhat ornate taste.

The Table of Contents came next, then the dedication "To the Very-Christian King of France and of Poland, Henri III." After a paragraph comparing the human body to the Kingdom of France, governed by the Gracious King, Paré explained to the King why he had written his book. A brief, liberal translation of this might be interesting; the original may be found in Malgaigne, I, p. 1-6.

> For more than forty years I have worked for the clarification and perfection of the Art of Surgery, striving for two things especially, that the ignorant do not debase it by relegating it to a mechanical art, and in this work I have aimed that the Ancients from whom we came should surpass us only in the development of principles, and (said without envy or offense) that posterity should surpass us only by the addition of their own inventions. I have been prodigal of myself, my toil and my facilities, not sparing time, working night and day, nor my freshness. I have used a great deal of money required to produce so laborious and important a book, for use of poor

scholars. These, instructed in theory, were chilled, finding neither the means nor the way to practice the science they had learned.

For this reason, putting aside other considerations and anticipating only the benefits to posterity and the illumination of France, I have done all I could for those who use it, to clear surgery of the crudeness of past centuries and the envy of those who profess it. I say I have clarified, strengthened and enriched it, not alone by virtue of what I write, but also with more than three hundred and fifty illustrations I have had drawn. I have included more than five hundred figures and pictures of anatomy and of instruments needed for surgery. Each of these has been properly titled and the use of each properly described, so the figures are not presented from vanity. Moreover, by the grace of God, I have included the works of other earnest men, rich in truth and experience and able to accomplish what they advise. To avoid presumption in my desire to publish this great book, I have consulted with many excellent men, physicians as well as surgeons, who encouraged me to proceed with it and to complete it. Some want to have it in Latin; I leave this to those who more than I have studied to learn it and have the leisure to do it. Some would like to use it in their schools to lecture to their pupils, wishing to share equally with me in the glory of bringing to foreigners something of which they have no acquaintance under the sun, who could neither operate dextrously nor teach perfectly, in the Kingdom your Majesty rules. Also I dare say without fear of being misunderstood, that I know no man so sensitive or so difficult to satisfy, who cannot learn something from this book. This applies to those who know the art of what they see, those who know surgery, as well as those who have had only ordinary experiences.

With all that, Sire, this is my master-piece, the accumulation of all the works of one of your old servants and subjects, that I thus dare to put at your Majesty's feet, as much to acknowledge the duty and service that I owe you, as for the honor you have been pleased to grant me, keeping me in your service in the capacity of your Premier-Surgeon. Here I have served under three Kings, predecessors of your Majesty, to whom I hope to make a remembrance of my faithful service and my very humble affection. By this means, I hope to strengthen this book to advance head erect through the universe, being honored by the favor of the greatest and most powerful Monarch of the world, who favored my past service and my fresh works presented here, not disdaining to overlook my faults. The late King Charles IX, of happy memory, prompted by your Majesty's Most-Serene Queen-Mother, who commanded me to publish these writings under the Royal Name, wished to see this book, promising that my labors and services would be remembered. Your Majesty will remember how many Princes and Great Lords I have served by saving their lives at your command, by the Grace of God and the careful use of my hand and experience in the art I profess. From King to King, my wish followed and my services continued, as from one Powerful King to another Invincible, I repeated my vows and dedicated my knowledge to the common good, assured that the Queen would keep her word to me and that the greatest King of the Universe would favor his humble servant and would support part of the burden on the surgeon grown old in the service of the House of France and would honor the frontispiece of this book with the happy and admirable name of Henri, a safeguard and defense to my honor, to prevail against the tongues of the envious and of calumnators. In my book, I have used no deceitful language, being careful that my words were proper and significant, bringing France the honor for which this book is designed; and dedicated to you, Sire, praying God to grant you for your contentment, long prosperity and perpetual happiness.

Your very humble and most obedient servant and subject,
A. Pare.

On the next few pages, Paré put his portrait: that of an old man with thin hair and a scant beard, his temporal arteries prominent and his eye weary. This is followed by poems written to him by his friends, including the great Court poet Ronsard. It may surprise some that Ambroise tried his own hand at poetry, but a sonnet written by the author is included. During his years at the Court, when the Kings sought recognition as protectors of the Muses, poets and writers flourished there, as did painters and sculptors. His writing shows evidence of progressive refinement and polishing of Paré's language; it is not unexpected that he was interested in the poet's technique and practice it himself under the guidance of the ablest men of the country. Its merit eludes me; I cannot translate the old French into a pleasing English form.

Then comes a section *Au Lecteur,* to the Reader, giving Paré's reasons for having written as he did. Here he is speaking, not to the King, but to his peers and again to the poor student trying to learn surgery, with few books written for him in his own language. Paré explained that his quotations from the ancients were included, not to steal from them, but to demonstrate the age of the knowledge he included and to show the additions in information that had come since they had written on the topics. Similarly, to benefit the reader, he did not hesitate to include the good works of contemporaries on subjects in which they were more expert than himself. In these cases he acknowledged his sources, so he might not be thought guilty of plagiarizing the works of others. Notwithstanding these quotations, he said, this was his own work, built on his own foundations and the edifice and materials were his own. He said that the physicians accused him of having gone beyond the limits of surgery in his writings, particularly concerning fevers. He pointed out that since Medicine and Surgery are parts of a whole, there is no clear cut boundary between them. The fathers of medicine had treated on both subjcts. He insisted that the surgeon must know fevers to practice surgery or the lives of his patients would be endangered. All the former great surgeons had included the topic in their writings and the subject hadn't changed. He admitted that the surgeon has much to gain from the help of the good physician, but in many instances he must work alone and the patient should not suffer from the surgeon's ignorance.

Again, Paré defended his writing in French, pointing out the examples of Hippocrates, Galen, the Arabs and others having written in their vernaculars. He added that he considered the French language as noble as that of any foreigner. Concerning the charge that the practice gives laymen a chance to learn the secrets of the profession, he expressed astonishment that men "who can learn the roads to the heavens, the movements of the sun and the moon and the dimensions of the earth" should not be permitted to know themselves and the marvelous construction of their own bodies. He had learned that sciences are composed of things, not words. The former are essential; words merely express and describe them.

When finally taking leave of the Reader, Paré reminds him that his life had been spent for his country, seeking always to advance the cause of the young surgical apprentice to whom his writings are addressed. He thanked God for having calling him to the practice of surgery, "the knowledge of which cannot be bought with money, but only with work and experience." This is true in all countries, he said, for the laws of medicine are not those of Kings or other rulers, but come from God, whom he prays will bless his work, which will glorify it eternally.

That Paré's book was popular can be judged from the fact that a new edition was demanded so quickly that all the laborious details of rewriting, editing, preparation of new wood-cuts and printing were completed four years later. The first edition must have received hard usage too, for Malgaigne could find only one copy in existence in 1840, in the library of St. Geneviève, although Doe was able to locate twenty-one of them, with the better facilities of communication available to her.

Just two days after the litigation over his *Oeuvres* was heard in Parlement, Paré's new wife had her first baby. Anne Paré was baptized at St. André-des-Arts on 16 July, 1575. This was a truly splendid christening. The infant's godmother was the great Princess Anne d'Este, widow of François, late Duke de Guise, and mother of Henri, the present Duke de Guise. Now she was Duchesse de Nemours, having married Jacques de Savoy, Duke de Nemours and of Genoa, son of Philippe de Savoy, Paré's old enemy at Hesdin. The godfather was the eight year old Charles de Savoy,[123] son of Anne and of Jacques de Savoy (Le Paulmier, p. 93).

On 2 September, the King fell ill with a severe earache, which frightened him greatly, since his brother François II had died so. During the next few days the King did not follow the advice of his physicians, since a Carnival was going on. In addition to his heavy duties of the moment, he took little rest, spending his nights in exhausting parties. On 10 September, after a short ride, he returned with a severe earache and was so ill that his life was despaired of by all his physicians except Le Grand. The old rumor of Paré poisoning François II was revived and the surgeon was careful to do nothing except on the advice of and in the presence of his physicians (Paget, p. 199). Malgaigne (Intro., cci) noted that since their defeat by Paré over the publication of his book, the physicians were so jealous of him that they sought to exclude him from Court consultations. The King survived his otitis, but Paré's fight with the physicians continued for another ten years.

Meanwhile, the affairs of the Government wallowed in a sea of unrest. Fighting continued around the country; both factions lost faith in the irresolute Council, the vacillating Queen-Mother and the completely incompetent King. We have no record of Paré's reaction to the frivolities of his silly King. He probably considered this none of his business and remained as resolutely loyal to Henri III as he had been to his predecessors.

1567

In 1567, Ambroise became involved in a legal tilt with the College of St. Côme (Malgaigne, Intro., p. cclxxxvii). In order to take advantage of a bequest to the College made in 1574 by one of its late members, Nicolaus Langlois, the statutes of the College were revised in terms not consistent with the originals. Paré and four other members, Du Bois, Guillemeau, Le Gay and l'Arbalestrier,[124] refused to sign it, and the quarrel went before the Parlement. On 10 April, the Faculté de Médecine got into the proceedings and the Dean, Henri de Monantheuil,[125] had their attorney sit in on the suit, in case Faculté affairs should become involved (Le Paulmier, p. 95). Because of the refusal of the five members to sign the proposed new statutes, they were redrawn in their original form, with two new articles added to permit the College to comply to the terms of Langlois' bequest. The entire body of twenty-four members then signed the new form on 11 May, 1577.

On 30 May, 1576, Jacqueline Rousselet's second child by Paré, a son, was baptized and named Ambroise. The godfathers were Charles, Count de Mansfeld,[126] and Charles, Marquis d'Elbeuf.[127] The godmother was Paré's old friend from Turin days, Dame Philippes de Montespedon, Duchesse de Beaupréau and Princesse de la Roche-sur-Yon (Le Paulmier, p. 94). Ambroise's children now were being sponsored by the nobility, but even this was to no avail; this son also died in infancy in the following January.

1577

On 14 January, little Ambroise Paré was buried in St. André's church.

On 27 March, Ambroise appeared at the Châtelet to witness the marriage contract between his beloved niece Jeanne and the surgeon, Claude Viart. Although Paget (p. 194) said that Viart had been a pupil or assistant of Paré's for twenty years, no supporting evidence for the statement is given. Misled by Bégin, Malgaigne (Intro., ccxxvi) believed that Viart married Ambroise's sister. Ambroise mentioned Viart several times in his writings, but those which are dated were written after the wedding. Le Paulmier (pp. 96, 254 & 270) discussed Viart, but reported no such long-term association. He had practiced at Nantes, a town on the Loire between Angers and the Coast and now was living near the Parés on the Pont St. Michel next door to Ambroise's old friend Pierre de la Rue, the tailor (Le Paulmier, p. 97). Viart died sometime around 1583, only six years after marrying Jeanne.

In addition to Jeanne's dowry bestowed upon her by Ambroise in 1574, Paré gave Viart his long red surgeon's robe with velvet trimmings, all his surgical instruments, the blocks from which the illustrations for his *Oeuvres* was printed, costing him over a thousand écus, his books on the plague (1568), the *Five Books of Surgery* (1572), the *Two Books on Surgery* (1573) and those next to be printed, in Latin as well as in French. This gift seems to indicate that the Latin translation of his *Oeuvres* was already in process, since this is the only Latin edition that appeared. Paré reserved for his own lifetime the use of all these gifts.

Viart conferred upon his fiance a dowry of one hundred and fifty livres tournois and upon his death, all his clothes, luggage and jewelry. Should she die first, he was to recover his clothes, his arms and his horse, etc. (Le Paulmier, p. 254).

The newly married couple moved into their house in the Paré courtyard, but because of Viart's prolonged absences with the army in Flanders and Britany, the marriage contract was not legally registered until almost four years later (see 1581). Le Paulmier thought (p. 98) that Viart was away with the Duke d'Anjou on his expedition to the Low Countries in the autumn of this year.

On 31 October, Paré's old friend Philippes de Montespedon died. He had first served her husband, the Count de Montejan, in Turin. He had served her and her second husband, Charles de Bourbon, Prince de la Roche-sur-Yon, and she had been godmother to his second child by Jacqueline Rousselet only a little more than a year earlier. Many of the friends of his youth were being lost to Paré by death.

On 14 December, Paré had a master-mason come to inspect the courtyard house he had given to the Viarts. The mason described the windows looking into the court. The house was enclosed on the east and north sides by other existing buildings, so these windows constituted the only exposure of the Viart house to the sun and air. To protect them from possible later encroachment by other future acquirers of the Maison de la Vache, Paré went to his attorneys again on 19 December and bequeathed the Viarts perpetual rights to this exposure (Le Paulmier, p. 260). Occupied as he was with his practice, his Court obligations and the preparation of a new edition of his Oeuvres, Ambroise still had time to anticipate and try to forestall possible future trouble for his loved ones.

1578

The New Year of 1578 brought nothing new to the troubled affairs of France, but it brought a new baby to the Paré household. On 6 February, Jacqueline had her third child, Marie, baptized at St. André-des-Arts. The godfather was Jean Camus,

Sieur de St. Bonnet, Paré's lawyer, secretary of the King and Recorder of the Privy Council. On 31 August, 1570, he had been appointed Royal Comptroller of Finance, after having given the King a present of twenty-five thousand livres tournois (Le Paulmier, p. 98). One of the two godmothers was Marie de Tillet, wife of Pierre Seguier, Chevalier, Sieur de Sorel and Civil Lieutenant of the Provost of Paris. On 1 August, 1576, Seguier had succeeded his father as President of the Paris Parlement. The second godmother was Marie Boullaie, the infant's grandmother. Le Paulmier noted that she was a widow now; Jacqueline's father must have died within the past four years, since he was alive on 31 January, 1574. Little Marie did not have Royal godparents; they were rich bourgeoise and important politicians.

In 1895/6, M. Valet reported discovering in the registers of the church of St. André, preserved in the Bibliothèque Nationale, the following notation: *1578, March 21, baptism of Ambroise, son of Claude Viart, Surgeon of Paris and of Jeanne Paré. Godfathers: M. Ambroise Paré and Guillaume Loquet.* I have found no other reference to a child of Viart and Jeanne, although Le Paulmier, p. 115, reported that on 20 April 1589 Jeanne had a son François by her second husband, François Fôrest.

The first edition of Paré's *Oeuvres* apparently sold out rapidly, for despite all the work entailed, Ambroise had the copy ready for publication of the second edition in the spring of 1578. His original publication privilege was for nine years, but the Faculté had had its decree of 1535 reaffirmed by the Parlement on his last brush with them.

Gourmelen no longer was Dean of the Faculté, having been replaced by Claude Rousselet, probably related to Paré's wife. For these or possibly other reasons, Ambroise submitted the manuscript for their appraisal on 5 April, 1578, in the care of Dr. Guillaume Lusson, who in 1594 became Dean (Le Paulmier, p. 99). Noting that "this man" had conformed to the decree of Parlement granted them, the Faculté ordered "his heavy volume" examined and evaluated by a committee to report on 2 August. The committee consisted of Drs. Jean Liebault,[128] Michel Marescot, Duval, Pierre Lamer,[129] Jean Haultin,[130] Germain Courtin,[131]

Jean Martin,[132] Claude Rebors,[133] Giles Héron,[134] and Lusson himself (Le Paulmier, p. 99).

On 2 August, the committee met, but all members were not present. Those present decided to send their written opinions to the Faculté, which would make the decision regarding approval or rejection. The Commission was advised, moreover, that it would have to produce publicly works submitted for its examination, so it was decided that the book could be published after correction. The Faculté found that it could actually exercise its censorship only by printing the book. Paré passed it on to Gabriel Buon for publication; printing was finished in February of the next year.

1579

Despite his regrets over the matter, Ambroise had an actual advantage in not having had formal schooling in surgery: it forced him to rely upon his own observations. In instructing young surgeons, he quoted his personal observations widely. These make most interesting reading to get a feeling of the customs of the time. Some of the accounts are dated and hence can be correlated with Paré's age and general store of information.

On 1 February, 1579, Ambroise attended an autopsy and dissection in the Royal College of Surgeons. The specimen was the body of a twenty-one-year-old girl who had been hanged ten days after delivery for having killed her baby with her own hands. The dissection was done the day after the execution. Malgaigne (II, p. 666) translated a long Latin report of the case written by Dr. Severin Pineau,[135] one of Paré's friends. It describes the type of mass consultation and autopsy attended by interested medical men when they had the opportunity to try to answer perplexing questions. The report went into considerable detail concerning the doctors present and their methods of procedure.

The dissection was done in the presence of the Provost of the College, André Malezieu.[136] Jacques d'Amboise,[137] Master of Arts and Bachelor in Surgery, dissected the cadaver expertly and demonstrated the parts. This was an innovation; in Paré's youth this task was delegated to a low barber-surgeon. "Following the custom of the College," the visiting observers surrounded the autopsy table. Pineau listed them in the order of their arrival: Dean Robert Gaignard; Nicholas Langlois; François des Neux; Guillaume DuBois, King's surgeon; Ambroise Paré, King's Premier-Surgeon; Louis Le Brun; Jean d'Amboise, King's Surgeon and Surgeon of the Châtelet; Jean Cointeret, the Queen-Mother's Surgeon, also on the staff of the Châtelet; Nicole des Neux; Raol Le Fort; Richard Hubert, Pierre Pigray, Antoine Portail, Jacques Dionneau and Ismael Lambert,[138] all King's Surgeons; Jerome de La Noue,[139] Surgeon of the Queen-Mother; Pierre Cheval; Dr. Simon Piètre; Urbain l'Arbalestrier and Jacques Guillemeau, King's Surgeons. Also present were Louis Hubert and Philippe Collot, both Surgeons of the King-Elect, Josse de Beauvois and Claude Viart. There were two visiting surgeons from Montpellier whom Paré met on his visit there, Laurent Joubert, Physician and Royal Professor of the University, and Surgeon Bartholoméy Cabral. Also in attendance were some medical and surgical students and diligent anatomists who had been studying animal and human dissection for a year. Among them, if he was not mistaken, he noted, were P. Erald, Jérome Coupé, both from Champagne and Gaspard Bauhin of Bâle, then a very celebrated physician of his country and Professor-elect of Botany and Anatomy. Really, quite a distinguished gathering it was.

The doctors wanted to find out, first, if there is a connection between the descending mammary veins and the ascending epigastrics, to see if in a recently delivered woman the "blood by which the mother nourished their infants" comes from vessels around the uterus and other lower parts; whether the milk is produced by the uterus or whether the connection is via other vessels, etc. As Malgaigne noted, "such questions!"

The question then arose of whether the bones of the pelvic separate during delivery. The spectators were asked their opinions in advance; most of them thought not. They found then that by direct leverage on the intact extremities, the pelvis symphysis separated. By other manipulations, **they found that** the other pelvic joints, usually fused at this age, permitted motion. Although the demonstration was obvious, Pineau said that some "hardened their heads" and believed this a unique phenomenon, and not to be expected in the usual cases of delivery. Malgaigne was surprised that no one inquired whether this particular woman might not have had a malady of the synchrondroses independent of her post-partum state. Paré himself said that it was contrary to his previous belief and writings, but he saw it. He added that he would refer "those who wish not be believe it to the book of Nature, who does things we can't understand, especially that these bones do open and close at delivery" (Malgaigne, II, p. 668; Hamby, p. 100).

LES OEUVRES, SECOND EDITION

On 8 February, 1579, the last pages of the second edition of *Les Oeuvres de M. Ambroise Paré* came from Gabriel Buon's press and presumably were on sale a few days later. The format was the same as the original but somewhat larger, by one hundred and sixty pages and sixty-six wood-cuts. The illustrations were located about the same as in the first edition, but were duplicated and a set added in one section at the end of the text. Ambroise explained that he did this, "not minding the extra expense," so the King could examine the pictures without having to leaf through the book, thus saving time he might want to devote to more serious things. Paré's own unsigned and undated portrait was included just before his dedication to the King and again at the end of the section of isolated illustrations. His motto, "Labor improbus omnia vincit," roughly, "Unceasing work conquers everything," appeared at the end of the text.

The subject matter was not changed greatly, despite the admonitions of the Faculté. The section on Generation, considered indecent in the first edition, was left unchanged. Ambroise humored the Faculté by omitting the section on Fevers, but he did not omit the material. Instead, he divided it into parts which he included in appropriate places in the book on Tumors, to be sure the young surgeon would have it available when needed.

The *Book of Animals* and that on *The Excellence of Man* were new, as Doe (p. 113) noted; probably the result of Paré's wider reading, permitted by his greater leisure. *Of Venins* was greatly expanded in this edition; in the first edition this section was practically taken from that of the *Five Books of Surgery* of 1572. Doe remarked that the additions were from other authors, rather than from Paré's own experiences.

Another edition of the book has caused some speculation. It too is called the second edition, but is dated 1597. The title page bearing this date is not the elaborately engraved one of the 1579 edition; it simply was set up in type and printed. As Doe remarked, under such circumstances reversal of the last two numerals of the date would easily be overlooked. The text itself is that of the 1579 edition, while one of 1597 would have come between the fourth edition of 1585 and the fifth of 1598, both of which were much larger and more elaborate. It is more likely that this actually was a reissue of sheets left over from the original printing of the second edition. Doe was able to find only one remaining copy of this specimen, in the Library of the Académie de Médecine of Paris. She located seventeen copies of the original second edition.

On 8 October, Jacqueline Paré was baptized at St. André-des-Arts church. This was Jacqueline Paré's fourth baby. Her godparents were of the political gentry this time; the godfather was M. Jean Lallemont, Seigneur de Vousse, Master of Petitions and King's Councillor. The godmothers were his sister, Marie Lallemont, wife of M. Daubray, Provost of Merchants of Paris, and Antoinette Lallemont, wife of Pierre Charles, King's Auditor and Councillor in the Chamber of Accounts.

1580

During the summer of 1580 the constantly endemic plague, which had been smoldering for two years, burst into renewed vigor in Paris. Sixty thousand people died in the city between June and November. When a major epidemic seemed to be developing, the merchants of the city and the Provosts of Paris met to plan means of combating it. The Faculté de Médecine was consulted. The Dean, Henri de Monantheuil, apparently was responsible for including Paré in the Council. On 12 June,

Paré was granted a privilege for printing a sort of a handbook of plague treatment. Fortunately, sheets printed for the 1568 *Traicté de la Peste* were available. By revising the titlepage and rewriting the introductory material, Paré had the copy ready for Buon to issue the new book quickly. He dedicated it to "Messieurs les Provosts des Marchans & Eschevins de ceste ville de Paris," along lines used in the earlier dedication to Castellan, saying that he had condensed this book from his works to help the city beset by the plague; the book could be bought and carried more easily by young surgeons than could the more costly and heavier volume of his *Oeuvres*.

New measures were developed for handling the epidemic, including segregation of the patients. Provision had to be made for the care of a large number of them. On 3 July, Dean de Monantheuil, Ambroise Paré, the Provost of Paris and an architect visited the Faubourgs St. Marcel and St. Victoire. On 7 July, de Monantheuil, two court lawyers, the Civil Lieutenant, the Provost of Merchants and the Abbé of St. Geneviève inspected the village of Grenelle and marked out the plan of buildings to be erected there. This was the origin of the "maisons de peste" or pest-houses, as the term has persisted to the present.

Most of the Parisians who could afford it moved out of the city. Physicians and surgeons were importuned to remain and care for the poor and unfortunate sick. It is interesting to find that the late Faculté Dean, Etienne Gourmelen, was "called out of the city" at the time. This explanation was given on 12 February, 1581, in a twenty-eight-page pamphlet he issued containing the Faculté's advise on the management of the epidemic. The Faculté's Register noted that the greatest of the physicians deserted the city and did not return until just before the epidemic began to subside (Doe, p. 61).

At about this time also appeared Gourmelen's own book on surgery, *Chirurgicae artis, ex Hippocrates, cum aliorum veterum medicorum decretis . . . Libri, III, Paris, 1580*. In this he castigated Paré for his use of the ligature in amputations. He considered the cautery vastly superior. As Doe said (p. 25), the book was "an idiotic appeal to authority and tradition; the very thing Paracelsus[140] would have loved to burn." Unfortunately for Gourmelen, but fortunately for posterity, this book stung Paré into a fury of resentment against this pedant who would not let him alone. This was the final stimulus required for him to begin now writing the *Apologie, et Traicté Contenant les Voyages Faicts en Divers Lieux* (*Apology, and Tract containing the trips made to different places*), to go into the fourth edition of his *Oeuvres*.

M. Christophe Jouvenel des Ursins[141] was Lord of Chapelle-Gautier, of Doüe and of Armenonville, Marquis de Trainel, Governor of Paris and Lieutenant-General of the Ile-de-France, Chevalier of the Order-of-the-King and Councillor of the King's Privy Council, a very important person. On the last day of August 1580, he was riding between Chaalis and Armenonville, about forty-four kilometers from Paris, when his huge war-horse capered and fell upon him, driving his back into the rough gravel. The horse, being a brave one, at once attempted to get up, but slipped in the loose footing and fell heavily upon his master again. The Lord was unconscious. His life probably was saved by a companion who dismounted and dragged him away from the floundering horse. M. des Ursins was put to bed in his house. His wife called for surgeons from Senlis and Dampmartin. The widow of the late Constable Montmorency sent the King's Surgeon-in-Ordinary, Pierre le Fèvre, who happened to be at Chantilly at the time. He bled the Lord and treated him for the injury, but was alarmed at the blood suffusing under the skin of the back and down into the abdomen and thighs. He sent for Paré.

Ambroise described the incident (Malgaigne, III, p. 468; Hamby, p. 143) saying, "For the service I owed you and all your house, I promptly mounted horse." He incised the skin of the lower back to evacuate the clot, and serum drained so profusely for ten or twelve days, "I began to fear your whole body might melt, leaving you tabetic." He considered it necessary to make other incisions to drain the large cavities. Although he was the King's Premier-Surgeon and enjoyed more authority on injuries of this type than perhaps did anyone else in the world, he told the family he wanted consultation. Madame des Ursins promptly sent an appeal to the King for Antoine Pigray, who was dispatched immediately. He also sent Drs. de Mouron and Haultin of the Faculté and surgeons Cointeret and Le Fort.[142] They came, examined the patient and, in consultation, agreed with Paré's proposal. The new incisions were made, the cavities drained and the patient began to mend. During his convalescence he and Paré discussed many matters. Among other things, M. des Ursins wanted to know why he had not been treated with mummy at the time of his injury. This particular nostrum was one of Paré's pet aversions among the revolting pharmacopeal items in use at the time. He explained this to the nobleman in his own forceful style. This so impressed the Lord des Ursins that he urged Paré to put the story into print. Educated Gentlemen then knew a great deal of what was known of medicine, being responsible for the welfare of hundreds of underlings, and M. des Ursins thought they should be disabused on this subject. Although he was about to have the Latin edition of his *Oeuvres* published, was revising the second edition to publish the fourth and was writing his *Apologie, et Traicté*—for all that, Paré also enthusiastically took on this new assignment and had it published within two years. Although he was seventy years old, Paré certainly could not be accused of slowing down!

1581

On 12 February, 1581, Catherine Paré, fifth child of Ambroise and Jacqueline, was baptized at St. André. Her godfather was M. Vincent Moussey, Councillor of Parlement. The godmothers were Barbé Rousselet, presumably an aunt, wife of Didier Martin, an archér of the King's Bodyguard, and her own half-sister, Catherine Paré, now twenty years old. This daughter Catherine was to be with Ambroise through the rest of his lifetime. She was to be married in this same church on 29 September, 1603, to Claude Hédelin, advocate, poet and Government official (Paget, p. 195).

A week after the baby was born, Ambroise had another stimulus to speeding the writing of his *Apologie*. On 18 February, the booksellers had on their shelves the essay on the plague that Gourmelen had written to tell how the disease should be handled. Apparently, he wrote best at a distance from the scene.

Between having children, writing and practicing, Ambroise was to have a new experience. On 28 March, his twenty-year-old daughter Catherine, sole survivor of his first wife's three children, was married (Le Paulmier, p. 101-104). The bridegroom was François Rousselet, brother of Catherine's stepmother. He was Secretary and Treasurer of the King's brother, the Duke d'Anjou. This Catherine was the one who most piqued the interest of Paget (p. 196), that gay romantic, who wondered why Claude Viart, four years earlier, had married her cousin Jeanne and not her. Perhaps it was something as simple as the possibility that a twenty-two-year-old woman appealed more to him than did a girl of sixteen. The newly-married couple may have had as little time for their honeymoon as had Ambroise and Jeanne Mazelin for theirs. In June, the Duke d'Anjou was off to the Netherlands again on one of his repeated attempts to carve out for himself a kingdom in the Low Countries.

In the section of his *Oeuvres* on Generation, Paré had expressed definite opposition to delivery by Caesarian section. As Doe (p. 113) remarked, this indirectly stimulated the writing of the best, and perhaps the first book on the subject in the 16th century. Paré's friend, François Rousset, disagreed with him and wrote a book, *Traitté nouveau de l'hysterotomokie ou enfantement Caesarien, Paris, 1581.* Henri de Monontheuil wrote at its end, "I have read this book, of which the discovery regarding the delivery called Caesarian seemed to me so well proved by reason and experience that I have judged it worth being made public." Ambroise was one of the witnesses to the affidavit.

The Latin edition of Ambroise's *Oeuvres* was ready for publication by his friend and pupil, Jacques Guillemeau. Guillemeau was born at Orleans in 1550 into a family of surgeons (Le Paulmier, p. 75). He was educated as a classical scholar and then went into training with Paré. He lived in the Paré home for eight years, although we do not know just when. Ambroise made this statement himself in a long poem he wrote to Guillemeau, included in the latter's *Tables Anatomiques* published in 1586. The poem was reprinted by Doe (p. 83) to make it available to modern readers. Guillemeau served under Paré at the Hôtel-Dieu and went with him to the wars. He became Surgeon-in-Ordinary to Kings Henri III, Henri IV and Louis XIII. He was appointed Provost of the College of Surgeons in 1595. Le Paulmier considered his best work to be *l'Heureux Accouchement, Paris, 1609*, in which he described saving the life of Paré's daughter Anne Simon in 1599 by inducing labor, by a method he had learned from Ambroise. He also wrote in 1586 the best Renaissance book on diseases of the eye. Jacques died on 13 March 1612. His son Charles, born in 1588, became a physician in 1626 and was Dean of the Faculté in 1634/35.

Conforming to all the requirements, Guillemeau submitted his manuscript to the Faculté on 21 December 1581. As Paget remarked, that body seemed determined to prove itself a collection of asses. They became enraged, contending that the translation had not been made by Guillemeau, but was the work of a physician of the school who had not been recognized; "This was really too much arrogance on the part of the surgeons, who are not capable of writing the first page in Latin." Guillemeau had not claimed to have translated the book, he simply was the editor. In his dedication to Marc Miron, Guillemeau had said very plainly that the translation was the work of a friend who, absorbed by his studies and public affairs, had done it on the condition that his name should not appear. Sixty years later, Guy Patin "was sure" he had identified the friend as Jean Haultin, and that he was not just a translator, but the real author. The Faculté demanded that the title of the book should be changed and they appointed a committee composed of Simon Piètre, Jacquart, Le Comte, Ellain, Claude Rebors and Michael Maréscot to make the change. The committee proposed the title: *Ambroisii Pareii premarii Regis chirurgi Opera latinitate donata a docto quodam viro: cura et diligentia Jacobi Guillemeau, Chirurgi Parisiensis*. This was sent to the printer, Jacques Du Puy on 30 December, 1581, with the written threat that if any part of it were changed, the book would be destroyed and the paper "put to vile usage."

Printers even then were an independent lot. Du Puy proceeded blithely to disregard these dire injunctions completely. Paget (p. 205) said the book was printed in Germany, but all the indications are that it was printed in Paris. Doe (p. 159) said that Jacques Du Puy seemed to have done well in his business in spite of having some of his books seized for heresy. He continued to print successfully and left his son Jacques a business of some pretensions.

1582

In January, 1582, the Latin edition of Paré's *Oeuvres* appeared, indicating that the printing had been finished before the text was submitted to the Faculté. It also appeared with the original title unchanged, as if in deliberate contempt for the Faculté's order: *Opera Ambroisii Parei Regis Primarii et Parisiensis Chirurgi. A Docto viro plerisque locis recognita: et Latinitate donata Iacobi Guillemeau Regii à Parisiensis Chirurgi labore & diligentia, Ad Clarissimum virum Marcum Mironem Regis Archiatrum dignissimum. Parisiis, Apud Iacobum Du-Puys, sub signo Samaritanae Cum Priuilegio Caesar. Majestatis, & Regis Christianis. M.D. LXXXII* (Doe, p. 153).

The title page bore an engraving of a well surrounded by six pillars bearing an elaborate cover with flanking copings. The well cover was in the form of a second circular, columnated and elaborately domed superstructure containing a figure. On the coping stood six nude female figures, each standing on a rectangular pedestal, each having symbols in hand. On the left of the wellcurb sat a draped female figure grasping the bail of the water bucket, which was suspended on a wheel attached to the roof of the well cover. On the right stood a draped, haloed male figure extending its right arm toward the seated woman. In front, on the slightly raised, curved pavement surrounding the wellcurb, stood two elaborately decorated, handled, narrow-necked vases resembling pedestaled amphori.

According to several critics, this Latin translation was made from the second French edition, but greater liberties were taken with the text. The translator altered, inverted and shifted various sections up to entire chapters. Doe noted that one unfortunate omission was the acknowledgment to the old friend of Paré's youth, Thierry de Héry, of quotation of material of *De la grosse verolle*, in which de Héry's text was followed almost verbatim. This inaccurate presentation was most unfortunate, since from this Latin text were made most of the other European language translations of Paré, including the English one of Th. Johnson in 1634. It was from numerous reprints of the Johnson translation that most of us English-speakers had our original introduction to Paré. Our mild elation over the feats of de la Rivière and of Paré in cracking the ironbound rules of the Faculté regarding medical publication in Latin alone must be tinctured with the realization of a concomitant great loss. The medical profession thereby lost the advantage of a universal language. On the favorable side was the immediate translation into Dutch, Italian, Spanish and English of sections of the book, making it available to the unlettered surgeons serving the armies and the people of these nations. In his dedication, Guillemeau said that, in service with the German and Spanish armies, he had seen their surgeons using as handbooks translated fragments of Paré's 1545 treatise on gunshot wounds, demonstrating to him the value of making Paré's surgery available to surgeons of other countries. This sparked the surgical renaissance for which Paré was responsible.

On 12 March, 1582, Ambroise was called to the house of the Lord Marshal de Biron to see M. Bernault de l'Estrelle, a Gentleman in his company (Malgaigne, III, p. 488; Hamby, p. 143). M. de l'Estrelle had been fencing with the Baron de Bouluet of Quercy, when the Baron's epée, tipped with an inch-wide, flat button, struck him in the left orbit. So violent was the blow that this blunt instrument drove through the orbit and face and down into the neck to the level of the fourth cervical vertebra. It did not break through the skin there, but left a black hematoma. Paré noted that the Baron was a strong and powerful man, which he must have been, since on the second attempt he jerked the sword tip out with its bulky button in place. The patient's head and neck swelled greatly and he could not turn his head. He was seen at once by M. Louis Paradis, M. de Biron's surgeon, and the army surgeon, Solin Crinel; they advised calling Paré. After examining the patient, Ambroise concurred with the attending surgeons' advice and bled him from the cephalic vein. They put pigeon's blood into the eye, for this was esteemed as a true eye balm. They incised the black area where the sword tip had approached the skin of the neck, draining a large amount of blood, deflating the swollen head and neck. They cut off the patient's hair and put plasters over the head and neck. The attendants were astonished that the patient retained his vision. Pigray, Cointeret, le Fort, Dionneau, Viart, Nicolas Marc, and other physicians and surgeons visited him to see the wound treated. Paré concluded his account: "He was cured, thanks to God, in twenty-four days and without losing any bone fragments, which is most remarkable. If asked to explain it, I should say that perhaps the displaced orbital bones could have been replaced as the epée was withdrawn."

On 7 June, Paré was called to treat a child in the rue St. Denis (Malgaigne, III, p. 489; Hamby, p. 147). The twenty-six-month-old son of Mathurin le Beau, a merchant milliner living at the sign of the Silver Crown, was playing in the street when the wheels of a coach loaded with five Gentlemen ran over his body. People screamed at the coachman, who stopped his horses and in pulling up, they backed the coach wheel over the baby's body again. The child was carried into his father's house. Believing him to be dead and evicerated, the family called Paré. Ambroise examined the infant carefully and could find no sign of fracture or dislocation. He sent someone to an abattoir at the city gate to get a freshly removed sheepskin. He rubbed the baby's body with oil of roses and myrtle and wrapped him naked in the warm sheepskin. The youngster must have been awake by then, for Paré said he gave him oxycrate[143] to drink, instead of mummy; this account was written in his book on that subject. He had the mother keep the child awake for the next four or five hours "so the blood would not so much run to the interior of the body." Over the next few days, he applied fomentations to reduce the contusions. He found then that the child could not stand or walk and was very constipated. He called in consultation the physician Simon Piètre, and he ordered some medication. Paré said that he feared a spinal injury, since patients so injured retain their excrements, while others have no control of them. Since he had not found the cause of the palsy and "knowing that two eyes see more than one," he called in Jacques Guillemeau and Jean Cointeret, whom he called "as well-experienced in surgery as there are in Paris." The consultants found nothing new, so the treatment was continued and "in the end he was healed, thanks to God. He walked as well as he did before he was hurt."

A week later, on 16 June, Ambroise had his friends together to see another interesting patient (Malgaigne, III, p. 681; Hamby, p. 156). Marie d'Hostel was the twenty-eight-year-old wife of Pierre Herue, esquire of the kitchen of Mme. the Duchesse d'Uzés, and lived in the rue des Verbois beyond St. Martin-of-the-Fields, at the sign of St. John's Head. She had suffered from caries of the ankle, tibia and fibula for three years and at last the pain became intolerable. Amputation was decided upon. Master Barber-surgeon Jean Charbonnel was going to do it, using Paré's ligature method of hemostasis instead of the cautery. The Faculté physician, Jean Liébault, was there, with the surgeons Claude Viart, Mathurin Heron and Paré. Ambroise reported that Charbonnel made his incision and divided the bones four inches below the knee. He caught the vein, then the artery, with the pincer-like hemostatic forceps called the crow's beak, and tied them. Paré reported that during the rapidly performed operation, not a pallet (approximately five ounces) of blood was lost. Paré advised Charbonnel to let more flow, since Hippocrates had found it good to let such wounds bleed well before suturing, to prevent inflammation.

It is interesting also that this is the last dated appearance of the name of Claude Viart. He died sometime between this episode and 1584, leaving Jeanne Paré a widow.

A point of interest in these old case reports is the eagerness with which physicians and surgeons of the period assembled to watch the work others were doing. Dozens of men of all ranks, from Professors and King's surgeons to barber-surgeons' apprentices crowded the anatomical theatres and autopsy rooms, as well as the patients houses. When an unusual case developed, the surgeon's friends came to watch his methods of therapy and to observe the outcome. Perhaps this was because books were so scarce and of such comparatively poor quality that surgeons as well as doctors had to learn by observation. If the theories of the day were unsatisfactory, they could at least see action and effect. The number of consultations is a little surprising also. It is doubtful that these people were less sure of their excellence than those of the present, or that they valued the suggestions of others any more than do men nowadays. Probably, the penalty for failure without adequate sharing of responsibility was greater than one could bear alone. Humble as Paré expressed himself before God and his superiors, his single-handed tilts with the Faculté de Médecine prove that he did not underestimate the value of his own knowledge of his subject in relation to theirs. It is likely that his great love for teaching led him to gather his peers as well as the poor young surgeons around him, whether or not he hoped for any real help from them.

On 23 August, 1582, Paré obtained his ten-year privilege for publication of his book on mummy, promised to M. des Ursins two years earlier. It must have gone on sale before the end of the year, since in January of 1583 a pamphlet written by an anonymous author appeared attacking it.

This little book of seventy-five pages of text, with twelve woodcut illustrations was entitled *Discours d'Ambroise Paré, Counseiller et Premier Chirurgien du Roy. A scauoir, De La Mumi, De La Licorne, Des Venins, Et De La Peste. Aves une table des plus notables matiers contenues esdits Discours. A Paris. Chez Gabriel Buon, au clos Bruneau, à l'ensigne St. Claude. 1582. Avec Privilege du Roy.* Much of the book was included in the fourth edition of his *Oeuvres* and may be found in Malgaigne, III, p. 468.

This book contains a splendid copper engraving of Ambroise. His hair was thinner now, his face more lined and his beard a little longer; but the eyes were bright and shrewd. The temporal arteries were more prominent than before, as is natural, since an insert in the upper left corner bears the surgeon's age, seventy-two years, and the date 1582.

This book was dedicated to "the very wise and powerful Lord, Messire Christofle des Ursins." In it, Paré recounted M. des Ursin's injury and his inquiry about why he had not been given mummy afterward. Paré replied that this would have done him more harm than good, and that the popular unicorn's horn was in the same category. He reminded Lord des Ursins that the ancient Jews, Arabs, Chaldeans and Egyptians had not embalmed their peoples' bodies to be eaten later by Christians, but out of hope of a new life after death. He described the process of embalming, with costly gums and spices for the rich and tar and pitch for poor, and commented on the funeral customs that prevented proper embalming of modern kings. He told of the body of a criminal he had obtained from the Criminal-Lieutenant Seguier, dissected and embalmed so well that twenty-seven years later it remained well preserved. He indicated that getting true Oriental mummies was a costly business and that defrauding merchants in this, as in other fields, were not averse to turning a dishonest livre by substituting counterfeit material. Thus the credulous patient might well be getting maggot-riddled, poorly-pickled, French criminal cadaver flesh not long off the gallows instead of the real article.

When Guy de la Fontaine, the celebrated physician of the King of Navarre, was going to Egypt and Barbary, Paré had asked him to look into the mummy and unicorn situation on their home grounds. In 1564, in Alexandria, the story went, there was a Jew who did a tremendous business in mummies. Dr. la Fontaine visited him and wanted to see his stock. This request was granted easily. The merchant opened a store room where many bodies were piled one on another. Asked whence they came, and if from ancient tombs, the Jew laughed heartily and said that he had prepared all of them himself within the last four years: they were the bodies of slaves or of any other cadavers he could find. On questioning, he admitted that they might have died of serious diseases, leprosy, syphilis and the plague; it made no difference to him how or of what they had died, as long as they were dead. Young or old, male or female, one couldn't tell such things after they had been embalmed. The Jew marvelled that Christians should be so greedy as to eat dead bodies. He told how he embalmed them, wrapping them in old linen bands, etc., to fool the Christians into believing that they were getting ancient material. Finally, la Fontaine told the Jew that the Christians were deceived into believing that they got mummies from ancient Jewish sepulchres. The Jew responded that it was impossible for Egypt to supply the demand for thousands of bodies, since the old mummifaction techniques had not been used for years.

Paré then wrote of the cases in which mummy was supposed to be the best remedy, such as M. des Ursins' own, that of M. d'Estrelle and the le Beau baby, and suggested how such injuries should best be treated.

On the subject of the unicorn's horn, Paré discussed the mythologic beast and described how the identity had been conferred upon the horn of the narwhal, that of the rhinoceros, and finally upon the elephant's tusk and ordinary bone. He discussed testing allegedly potent unicorn's horn again their fables: a scorpion would not cross out of a ring drawn on a table with water in which such a horn was soaked, or that a toad or other venomous animal would die if exposed to much of such water (Malgaigne, III, p. 505; Hamby, p. 148). Paré had experimented and found that the animals would cross such watery circles repeatedly, apparently not noticing them. Also, he had put a toad into water in which such a horn was submerged and after three days the toad "was as gay as the day he was put into it." He told of an honest merchant woman who had such a piece of "unicorn's horn" attached to a silver chain, hanging in a pitcher of water (Malgaigne, III, p. 506; Hamby, p. 149). Out of the goodness of her heart she would give the water to those who asked for it. One day a poor woman asked for some of the water to give her child, whose face was covered with a rash. The treated water had all been given away, but being a kindhearted woman and hating to disappoint, she gave the woman some ordinary river water. Ten or twelve days later the poor mother returned to thank the merchant woman for her kindness; the child was completely cured.

Paré continued then to hold these supposed cures up to ridicule, quoted authorities, told ridiculous stories of the gullibility of people who used such things and, in general, laughed the nostrums out of serious consideration. He ended, "That is how the unicorn's horn impresses me. If anyone can prove otherwise, I beg him to present it to the public and to consider my writing well intended."

1583

In January of 1583 appeared an anonymous attack on Paré's *Mummy, etc.* Entitled *Response au discours d'Ambroise Paré, touchant l'usage de la licorne,* the book was inscribed as read and approved by M. Grangier, Dean of the Faculté de Médecine. The author said that Paré did well enough in surgery, but when he crossed the boundary into the realm of medicine and pharmacy, "the little children mock at him." Paré was accused of translating Jordanus' book on plague and of presenting it as his own. Doe (p. 79) pointed out that Paré's plague material was published in his first *Traicté de la Peste of 1568,* while Jordanus' book did not appear until 1576.

Paré was accustomed to such *Responses* to his writings; in fact he had a few replies in preparation at the moment, but he began work on a *Replique* to this one. It would appear in the next year. Apparently, it required as long to get a pamphlet published then as it does now to get an article into a modern medical journal.

On 8 November, Ambroise proudly carried a new son into St. André's church for baptism. This was Jacqueline's sixth and last child. It was the fourth son for Ambroise; none of the three others had lived. For the second time, he named his little boy Ambroise. One godfather was M. Jacques Maréschal, King's Councillor, Procurer for his Majesty, Grand Provost of France and Advocat for the State Council. The second godfather was Paré's old friend and intimate, Jacques Guillemeau. The godmother was Anne de Mamères, daughter of M. Estienne de Mamères, Advocat of the Grand Council. Sadly enough, this son shared the fate of his earlier brothers; he was buried in the same church the following August. Of his nine children, only three remained; Catherine, wife of François Rousselet; Anne, aged eight years, and the second little Catherine, now two years old.

Ambroise remained at his post as King's Premier-Surgeon. He still attended his practice, although he delegated a great deal of the physical work to his assistants. Among the case reports submitted in the *Apologie* to bolster his claims for the superiority of the ligature, he reported the case of Toussant Posson, who lived at Beauvais, near Dourdon (Malgaigne, III, p. 682; Hamby, p. 158).

The patient had an ulcerated leg, the bone of which was exposed and which gave him frightful pain. After preparing him, Paré had the leg removed four inches below the knee cap by Daniel Poullet, one of his assistants, to teach him to do such surgery. Poullet tied the vessels very dextrously to stop the bleeding, without using the cautery, in the presence of Guillemeau and Jean Charbonnel. During convalescence, the patient was seen by Drs. La Fillé and Courtin, of the Faculté. Paré noted that the operation was done at the house of Jean Gohel, an innkeeper at the sign of the White Horse at Greve. He remarked also that since the man was poor, the Princesse de Montpensier paid for his board and room. "He was cured, thank God, and returned home with a wooden leg."

A week later, with le Fort and Le Noüe, Paré witnessed another such amputation performed by Antoine Renaud, a barber-surgeon, on Nicholas Nesnager in rue St. Honoré and recorded it (Malgaigne, III, p. 682; Hamby, p. 159). This case also had a good outcome.

Sometime this year Claude Viart died, leaving Jeanne Paré a widow. We have a reproduction of Jeanne's signature represented by Le Paulmier, p. 274, a court receipt for some money paid by François de Vigny. Viart had worked with Paré, had witnessed many of his recorded operations and had lived with Jeanne in the house in Ambroise's courtyard for ten years. Whether Viart left any living children is unknown. The only suggestion on the subject is the report by Valet that Paré stood godfather for an infant of Viart's named Ambroise. At any rate, Jeanne seems to have been a favorite of Ambroise's and she probably remained in her old home.

1584

In 1584 appeared Paré's little seven-paged pamphet: *Replique d'Ambroise Pare, Premier Chirurgien du Roy à la Response faicte contre son Discours de la Licorne.* This answered last year's anonymous attack upon his book on *Mummy*, etc. Against the accusation of having plagiarized others' writings, Paré pointed out that he had always tried to acknowledge the sources of his borrowed information and had taken the trouble to list them in his *Oeuvres*. It was here that he mentioned having spent more than a thousand écus to have his illustrations engraved. He answered his attackers' accusations carefully, reasonably and calmly. To his opponent's remark that it is better to err with the wise, Paré replied, "On the contrary, I would prefer to be alone in the right rather than to be in the wrong, not only with the wise but with the rest of the world." Finally, he humorously asked this attacker, "if he wishes to argue my reply, to omit the animosities and treat the old fellow more gently."

On 19 August, Ambroise and Jacqueline returned once more to St. André-des-Arts church, this time to bury the last of Paré's four sons, the eight-month-old Ambroise II. This was the last time he would experience this sad duty; the next family funeral he would "attend" would be his own.

At this time, Paré was completing the revision of his *Oeuvres* for the fourth edition. He had consulted with a Dr. Cappel, whom he described as a wise and widely-read Regent physician of the Faculté, about finding a doctor who knew Greek, to translate a section on diseases of the eye for his book (Malgaigne, II, p. 413). Apparently, this work was in progress but was not complete when the edition went to press. It contained only an elaborate table, taken from Galen. The completed section appeared in the fifth edition published post-humously in 1598, largely from Paré's own corrections.

1585

On 13 April, 1585, Gabriel Buon completed printing of the fourth edition of Paré's *Oeuvres* This was the greatest edition of them all, and the last that Ambroise saw through the press. Its title page was identical with that of the second edition except for specific numerical revisions. The place of the third edition is assumed to have been filled by the Latin *Opera* of 1582, published by Guillemeau.

A portrait of the author was printed from a copper engraving. Several of these were executed about this time, all based on that of Étienne (Stephanus) Delaulne[144] made for the 1582 *Discours de la Mumie*. Doe (p. 120) noted that various copies of this edition contained portraits by Giullis Horbeck or by A. Vallée.[145] In her own copy, the Vallee portrait was an obvious later insertion, while she considered the Horbeck the original illustration. These portraits were discussed by Le Paulmier (p. 136) who did not mention that of the fourth edition, but attributed the Vallée engraving to the fifth (1598) and the Horbeck to the sixth (1607) edition. Power said that Vallée's bust was drawn for the 1585 edition and that Horbeck's was based on it. In 1923, Haberling discussed the various portraits that later were published; he concluded that only those copied from Delnaulne were truly representative of Paré in his old age. While considering Paré portraits, Le Paulmier (p. 133) described and reproduced as the frontispiece of his book a 60 x 46 cm oil painting of a distinguished looking old gentleman. This painting was in the possession of Mme. la Marquise Le Charron, at the Château de Paley. It was dated 1575 and was entitled "Ambroise Paré, Premier Chirurgien du Roy." Le Paulmier considered it authentic; to me it bears little resemblance to the man figured in Paré's books. In 1929, D'Arcy Power described a portrait presented to the Royal College of Surgeons of England by Lord Berkeley Moynihan. It was copied in Paris from the original at Fecamp, attributed to Miereveldt. The dress and beard style date it to the first quarter of the 17th century, so it could not have been contemporary.

Ambroise had edited this edition carefully and added some one hundred and thirty pages to that of five years earlier. The *Discours de la Mumie* was included in the section on Contusions, and his *Replique à la response faicte contre son Discours de la Licorne* was added to that on Venins. These improvements and refinements no doubt were welcomed by the reader of his day, but what makes this edition really sparkle for the modern student is its inclusion of the *Apologie, et Traicté Contenant Les Voyages Faicts en Divers Lieux*. The annoyance of years of carping criticism by the tradition-encrusted Faculté finally boiled to the surface as the seasoned old surgeon sat down, pen in hand, to put the weight of his experience in the balance against the quotations of ancient authority by arm-chair philosophers.

He proved himself adept at his adversaries' own game; he quoted excellent authority for his own stand on controversial subjects. But much more effective was the story he told of how he proved his points by empirical evidence at the bedside, on the battlefield, in the charnelhouse and the anatomical theatre. It apparently galled him to have Gourmelen write that he would teach him (Paré) his lessons in surgery; this, Paré told his "petit maitre," he didn't think he could do. Paré pointed out with obvious pride that he had spent several years in the Hôtel-Dieu, learning surgery at first hand. Then, he proceeded to recount serially his experiences with the army, describing specific incidents that illustrated his points and naming responsible witnesses who could verify his statements.

His contempt for his adversary was scarsely concealed at some points; for example, when he described the terrible wounds suffered at the siege of Hesdin. He commented dryly that had "my little master" been there with his hot irons, "I believe they would have killed you like a calf for your cruelty." His readers probably smiled at the memory of Gourmelen's flight from the city during the plague, when at the end of Paré's description of the trip to Dourlan he remarked, "Here I will say nothing of my little master who was more comfortable in his house than was I at the war." Paré told how he had learned fortuitously that soothing dressings were better for gunshot wounds than was the cruel hot oil treatment previously used, and how he had had the strength of his conviction to adopt the new idea after experience had proved its superiority. In the case of the controversial use of the ligature to replace the cautery for control of amputation hemorrhage, he told how he had discussed the idea with other surgeons who agreed that it should be put to the test. He then described an impressive series of cases so treated, not by himself alone, but also by others he had taught, again listing witnesses. He livened and lightened the otherwise possibly heavy story with little touches of levity, as by describing the

Gentleman patient "going gaily home with a wooden leg," happy that he had been spared the ordeal of the hot irons.

These stories are of no clinical value to us now, but the clinical part of the account is not its sole interest; his description of the defense of Metz remains its most interesting historical account. Modern readers can only regret that Paré was not also provoked into extending his "diary" over a much wider field. Since so much of the history of that stirring era was written from hearsay, or colored luridly by the passions of partisan reporters, it is difficult for today's reader to evaluate properly those far-off motives and events. His dispassionate reports could have solved many tantalizing problems for us. Perhaps it is as well that he left things as he did. Otherwise, there might not exist the great urge to dig over old rubble in search of neglected gems. We would have welcomed especially more light on his own personal history and that of his family. Probably the thought never occurred to him that others later might be interested in him personally. He was fighting the cause of the advancement of his greatest love, Surgery. Sufficient for him was the accomplishment of his aim to teach young surgeons how to improve their treatment of the poor soldier, the object of his greatest compassion. Even after his clientele was composed largely of Counts, Dukes, Lords and Kings, he went into the dark hovels of Paris to bring the best of his art to the tailor, the fishmonger and the apprentice. Then, as now, this trait was the hallmark of greatness.

Characteristically, even after the appearance of this book, Gourmelen could not believe that he was beaten. Later in the year came a *Replique à un apologie publiee soubz le nom de M. Ambroise Paré, Chirurgien à Paris contre M. Estienne Gourmelen, docteur regent en la Faculté de Médecine,* an eighty-five-paged pamphlet written by B. Compérat, one of Gourmelen's pupils. It was an even more hysterical and stupid attack than the others had been. Paré had the grace to ignore it. No doubt Gourmelen's shade would flit more restlessly through the cypresses, could it realize that his only bid to a place in history lies in his unsuccessful attempt to defeat this ignorant and unlettered barber-surgeon.

In 1585, also appeared another book by Guillemeau, *Traite des maladies de l'oeuil, Treatise on Diseases of the Eye.* Garrison described this as decidedly the best renaissance book on ophthalmology. In 1958, a copy of the first Dutch edition by Abraham Dordrecht, Caen, 1597, was advertised by a New York book seller for $115.00. This book also contains a fourteen-line poem written in Guillemeau's praise by Ambroise. It has the flavor of expression of a father's praise for a beloved son.

Although Ambroise was successful in disposing of his professional enemy, he now was harassed by domestic strife. Apparently, he had got along well with his relatives, but his son-in-law, François Rousselet, began challenging Paré's trusteeship of his daughter's property. Rousselet claimed that part of the house Ambroise had given Jeanne Paré Viart should have gone to his own wife Catherine, on the death of her mother, Jeanne Mazelin. Other claims were made of misdirection of other funds, the total amounting to some twenty-seven hundred écus. This quarrel smouldered all through the winter.

1586

On 27 March, 1586, Ambroise and Jacqueline as one party and François Rousselet and Catherine Paré as the second, met in the Châtelet law offices of attorneys DeNets and le Camus. The complaint was outlined in detail (Le Paulmier, pp. 281-292). An agreement was made that Paré should settle the twenty-seven hundred écus on the party of the second part. On 14 May, Ambroise got an order from the King's Councillor and Provost of Paris, Antoine DuPrat, oldest son of the former Chancellor, voiding the previous settlement of the dispute. On 27 July, this paper was annoted with the indication that the action had been settled out of court to the satisfaction of both parties (Le Paulmier, pp. 293-295).

1587

Conditions in Paris continued bad. On 26 February, a man and a woman were burned at the stake in the Parvis Nôtre-Dame on the charge of witchcraft. Although a common form of execution in the Spanish-controlled countries, the French had been spared much contact with it, since the Inquisition had not been permitted to become established there.

On 1 March, news reached the people of Paris that their former Queen Marie, Queen of Scots, had been beheaded in London Tower at Elizabeth's order. Since she had always been a favorite of the French people, the news raised them to a fever of resentment. Public mourning was observed in the streets.

This had been a hard winter and it persisted into June. On 24 May, the vineyards in the neighborhood of Paris froze. Food sold at starvation prices. The authorities found it necessary to transport two thousand beggars from the city on 3 June to avoid having to feed them.

Ambroise must have been greatly depressed over the affairs of his country, and feeling the weight of his years. On 1 July, he made his will. To his two daughters by Jacqueline, Anne and Catherine, he left a house in the rue Garanciere in the Faubourgs St. Germain-des-Prés. To his assistant Denis Gaultier he willed his serge coat, his instruments and other goods, provided that Denis was still in his service at the time of Paré's death. Among his other possessions was listed a house at Ville-du-Bois, near Montlhéry, a strongly fortified town twenty-five kilometers from Paris on the road to Orléans.

No record has been found of Paré's acquisition of this property. Risch investigated the matter in 1933 and identified the place as the Grand Maison of the town. In 1580, the property belonged to François de Balsac d'Entragues,[146] who in 1579 married the late Charles IX's mistress, Marie Touchet. Risch supposed that Paré might have learned of the place while attending or even delivering Marie, although she did not marry François de Balsac until Charles had been dead for five years. At any rate, the house was left by Paré to his daughters Anne and Catherine jointly. In 1610, Catherine Paré Hédelin ceded her share of it to Anne Paré Simon (Le Paulmier, p. 129). Risch found that the Simons went into debt and the property was taken over in 1618 by a M. Thiboutot, who in 1623 sold it to a stranger for 9040 livres.

On 24 July, Ambroise first became a grandfather. It seems ironical that a man loving children as he did, and having sired nine of them, should be almost eighty years old before reaching this estate. Ironical again was the fact that this boon should have come from the one relative with whom he did not get along, François Rousselet. His daughter Catherine delivered a baby christened Florentine; Jeanne Viart was named godmother. Apparently, the family quarrel had been settled.

1588

On 11 January, 1588, Paré's niece Jeanne Paré Viart, now about thirty years old, married François Fôrest, a native of Orléans. The marriage contract had been drawn up on 29 December, 1587, with Ambroise and Francois Rousselet standing together as guarantors of her future. Fôrest was one of the King's Deputy Commissioners of the Châtelet and his supporters included several fairly influential political and military people (Le Paulmier, p. 296). The newly-married couple lived in the house Jeanne had formerly occupied with Claude Viart.

On 5 October, Catherine Rousselet gave Ambroise his second grandchild, a son they named Nicholas. The old surgeon was not very active now and he did not accompany the King to the meeting of the States-General at Blois, although he still held his commission as King's Premier-Surgeon. He was working against time, revising the fourth edition of his *Oeuvres* in preparation for the fifth, that would not be printed during his life time. By the time it would go to press in 1598, his loyal publisher Gabriel Buon would also have died and the book would be presented by his widow, Jeanne Rondel. This is the edition Malgaigne chose for his great production in 1840, although it is less authentically Paré's alone than was its predecessor.

At the meeting of the States-General at Blois, the King found that for all practical purposes, the Duke de Guise had control of the Government and that he had been reduced to the status of a figurehead. He had Guise assassinated on 23 December, 1588. On the following morning, the Cardinal de Lorraine was executed in a hallway by three of the King's halbardiers; none of his Gentlemen would accept the assignment. The Cardinal de Bourbon was kept under strict observation. The back of the Guise rebellion was broken. The bodies of the two brothers were burned; their ashes were thrown into the Loire.

News of the murders reached Paris on Christmas Eve. The Council of the Union met in the Hôtel-de-Ville; the Duke d'Aumale, brother of the late Duke de Guise, was appointed city Governor. The militia was put under arrest and the city gates were locked. A herald sent by the King was beaten and thrown out of the city. Public notice was posted that the League would enter into no negotiations with "Henri de Valois." Many other city and provincial governors followed suit. Only Blois, Tours, Saumur, Bordeaux and a few isolated spots remained loyal to the King. Beside himself with rage and frustration, Henri dissolved the States-General.

During these events, Paré had remained in Paris; Portail and Pigray were with the Court at Blois.

1589

On 8 January, 1589, at Blois, Catherine de'Médicis died in her bed of a terminal pneumonia. In the excitement of other events, the public was quite indifferent to her passing. Well-intentioned or malicious, her meddling was over. The people felt themselves well rid of her.

The Catholic League had chosen its way and would have nothing to do with Henri de Valois, King or not. Seeing mutual profit in collaboration, advisors of both sides gradually built up rapport between the King and Henri de Navare. The two agreed on a year-long truce in which Navarre would serve the King with complete faithfulness. The Huguenots would be protected from persecution. Navarre was given the town of Saumur, assuring him access to both sides of the Loire. On 30 April, the two Henris met at Plessis-les-Tours and made common cause in the attempt to reunite France. All Europe was electrified by the news promising internal French peace and unity. Philip II, who held himself the foremost champion of the Church, saw his plans crumbling. In May, the Pope informed Henri III that if the Cardinal de Bourbon and the Archbishop de Lyon[147] were not released within ten days, he would be excommunicated. He summoned the King to Rome to stand trial for the murder of the Cardinal de Lorraine.

On 30 April, Ambroise's niece Jeanne Paré Fôrest had her first son by her second husband and the baby was christened François. He died within a year. There is no evidence that the couple ever had another child.

Together, the King and Navarre made an effective force and in the main the people were glad to unite behind effective leadership. Toward the end of July, their army marched on Paris with forty-two thousand men, but found the city gates closed. After a parley, they laid siege to the city.

Henri III was installed in the home of the Count de Retz at St. Cloud, where Charles IX had paused temporarily during his mortal illness. This is on Paré's old road to Meudon. At eight o'clock in the morning of 1 August, a monk asked audience with the King, and despite the misgivings of his attendants, Henri saw him alone as requested. After handing the King a letter, the monk drew a knife from his sleeve and stabbed the King in the abdomen. His attendants rushed in and killed the monk with their swords. Henri was put to bed, his bleeding was controlled and he considered himself lucky. Portail and Pigray, in dressing him, however, found that the bowel had been pierced. In those days this carried a hopeless prognosis. The King's fever began mounting. Realizing that his end was approaching, Henri called Navarre to him and advised his followers to recognize him as King. He begged Navarre to return to the Catholic faith to unite the country behind him. About eighteen hours after his attack, the last of the Valois kings was dead. Portail did the autopsy and embalmed the body, in absence of his Chief.

Henri de Navarre was thirty-five years old, intelligent resourceful, witty and charming. Simple in bearing and manner, he was an excellent soldier and an inspiring leader. He could consider the different aspects of a problem and come to a quick decision. The Catholics offered him immediate recognition if he would abjure the Huguenot faith and return to the Church. It was beneath his dignity to accept the offer immediately, although his situation was precarious. He had barely two thousand Huguenots with him and, camped at Meudon, he humorously called himself The Highwayman. He sent Biron to administer the oath of allegiance to the mercenaries and the Huguenots, and he invited the Catholics who would to stay with him. He promised to consider their proposition thoroughly but he would not shift under pressure.

The League regained its confidence then. Realizing that he could not become King, the Duke de Mayenne proclaimed the Cardinal de Bourbon King and himself Lieutenant-Governor, a set-up the Duke de Guise had for so long planned and intrigued. Realizing that he would have to conquer his kingdom, Navarre marched on Rouen, and fought a shifting battle over the face of France. He again invested Paris on 1 November. Under the leadership of the Archbishop of Lyon, the League resisted strongly and threw him back. The year ended wtih the country still divided and Paris under siege.

1590

On January 4, Catherine Rousselet bore her third child, christened Charles, giving Ambroise his third grandchild.

The Committee of Sixteen, an official from each of the sixteen political divisions of Paris, was in full control of the city and by its overbearing policy, was gradually alienating the nobility, causing them to hold aloof, increasing Mayenne's difficulties. After Henri de Navarre had maneuvered around the Ile-de-France according to the needs of military pressure, in May he camped finally outside the city walls and prepared to starve Paris into submission.

Inside the city the food supply was quickly exhausted; famine prevailed. To divert and encourage the people the Church staged solemn processions and pawned the church plate for what food it would buy; the lot of private citizens became desperate. Violent demonstrations broke out within the city, demanding of the leaders "bread or peace." It was against this background that we have our last glimpse of Ambroise Paré, working as ever for the poor and helpless. Malgaigne (Intro., ccxciv) quoted l'Estoile's journal of the day:

> I remember that about eight or ten days at most before the siege was raised, M. de Lyon (the Archbishop), passing at the end of the Pont St. Michel, as he found himself besieged by a crowd of mean people, dying of hunger, who cried to him

demanding bread or death, and he not knowing how to dispatch them, encountered Master Ambroise Pare who said loudly to him, "Monseigneur, these poor people whom you see here about you are dying of the cruel rage of hunger, and demand pity of you. For God's sake, Monsieur, give it to them, if you would have God countenance you. And think a little of the dignity in which God has put you. The cries of these poor people which mount to heaven are a warning that God sends you, to consider the duties of your charge, for which you are responsible to him. Therefore, for this reason, and with the power we all know you have, get us peace, and give us wherewith to live, because the poor people no longer can do so. Don't you see that Paris perishes at the will of villians who wish to prevent the peace, which is the will of God? Oppose them firmly, taking in hand the cause of the poor afflicted people and God will bless and repay you."

Monsiegneur the Archbishop said nothing, or next to nothing, except that, contrary to his custom, he was patient to hear him out without interruption, and he said afterward that this good man had altogether astonished him, and again, that this was a different kind of politics than his own, but that he had awakened him and made him think of many things.

On Thursday, 20 December, 1590, on the Eve of St. Thomas, Ambroise Paré died in his house at the sign of the Three Moors in the rue de l'Hirondelle, at the age of eighty. He was buried on 22 December in the church of St. André-des-Arts, "at the foot of the nave, near the tower." The city gave him a "worthy funeral," but unfortunately no historian recorded the details (Packard, p. 126).

CHAPTER XI

L'Apostille, A Post-script

THE PARÉ FAMILY

AFTER THE DEATH of Ambroise, various members of the family left in court records evidence of minor difficulties in the settlement of his estate (Le Paulmier, p. 119). The name of his son-in-law, François Rousselet, appears prominently in these, suggesting that either he was an avaricious character or perhaps only a careful business man. The latter is probable, since he had been Treasurer of the King's brother, the Duke d'Anjou, and was that of the Queen of Navarre; such a role would be natural for him.

The widowed Jacqueline Rousselet lived on in the Maison de la Vache until her death on 26 June, 1600. She was buried the next day at St. André-des-Arts church (Le Paulmier, p. 122).

Only three of Ambroise's nine children survived him.

A. Catherine (1560-1616), the eldest daughter of Jeanne Mazelin, born on 30 September, 1560, was married in 1581 to François Rousselet, the brother of her step-mother. She had eight children, but nothing seems to be known of them except their names and details of their baptisms as recorded by Le Paulmier, p. 113. François Rousselet died before his wife and she returned to the Maison de la Vache to live until her own death on 21 September, 1616.

B. Anne Paré, first child of Ambroise and Jacqueline Rousselet, was baptized on 16 July, 1575, and presumably lived with her mother in the Maison de la Vache after her father's death. On 8 July, 1596, she was married to Henri Simon, King's Councillor and War Treasurer. They lived in the rue Prouvaires, in the parish of St. Eustace.

In 1599, according to Guillemeau, in his *L'Heureux Accouchement des Femmes,* Paris, 1606, she was rescued from a possible fatal hemorrhage (Le Paulmier, p. 120). Guillemeau's account, taken from Le Paulmier, reads:

> The year 1599, Madamoiselle (sic) Simon, still living, daughter of M. Pare, Councillor and First Surgeon of the King, being near term, was surprised by a great hemorrhage. She had known Madama La Charonne as Midwife, and was observed by M. Hautin, King's Physician-in-Ordinary and Physician in Paris, and M. Rigault, also a Paris Physician, because of attacks of syncope occurring every fifteen minutes from loss of blood. M. Marchant,[148] my son-in-law, and I were called. Finding her nearly pulseless, with feeble voice and blanched lips, I made the prognosis to her mother and her husband that her life was in great danger. The only way to save her was to deliver her immediately. I had seen this done by her father, the late M. Pare, who had me do it for a maid of Mme. de Santerre. The mother and husband entreated me to save her and put the case in our hands. Thus promptly, following the advise of Messieurs the Physicians, she was happily delivered of a lively infant.

Although the child was born healthy, it apparently did not live long, since in a legal document of 18 July, 1616, Henri Simon and Anne Paré were described as being childless (Le Paulmier, p. 121). No other descendants are recorded, nor is the date of Anne's death.

Le Paulmier (p. 129) attributed much of the worldly success of Anne's husband, Henri Simon, and of her brother-in-law, Claude Hédelin, to Anne's godmother Anne d'Este. By her second marriage, the latter was the wife of Jacques de Savoy, Duke de Nemours, and Hédelin was appointed Lieutenant-General of the baliwick of Nemours. Anne Simon seems to have loved her younger sister greatly. On 25 April, 1617, she and Henri Simon deeded to Catherine and Claude Hédelin Anne's share in the estate at Ville-du-Bois, left to them jointly in Paré's will (see p. 189).

C. Catherine (1581-1659), the last of Jacqueline Paré's

daughters, was married in the church of St. André-des-Arts on 29 September, 1603, to Claude Hédelin. Claude (1570-1638), a descendant of the noble family of Savoy, from which came the mother of François I, son of Jacques Hédelin, Esquire, and of Madeleine Bouvot, was sieur of Chauffoir, Montatelon and Bois-Regne. He was educated as a lawyer, was well-read and cultivated Latin and French poetry. He translated Ovid's *Heroïdes*. In Paris, he lived in the parish of St. Germain-le-Viele in la Cité. In 1610, seven years after their marriage, the couple settled at Nemours, family seat of the Duke de Nemours, fifteen kilometers south of Fontainebleau, and Claude was made Lieutenant-General of the baliwick in 1614. Le Paulmier (pp. 122-129) devoted a great deal of attention to this branch of the family and found valuable records and an oil painting of Ambroise Paré in the archives of the Château de Paley.[149] He reproduced (p. 124) a letter written by Catherine Paré Hédelin to one of her children.

Claude Hédelin and Catherine had twelve children, described in some detail by Le Paulmier. The most noteworthy perhaps was the first, François (1604-1676), who after being educated for the bar, became an ecclesiastic. Cardinal Richelieu entrusted him with the education of the Duke de Fronsac and gave him the Abbaye d'Aubignac, in the diocese of Bourges and that of Miemac, diocese of Limoges. Fronsac gave him a lifetime pension of four thousand écus.

In 1645, The Hédelins obtained the use as a family sepulchre of the Chapel of St. Peter in the church of St. Jean-Baptiste in Nemours. Here are buried Claude and Catherine; Claude's mother, Madeleine Bouvot; and the Hédelin children, the Abbé d'Aubignac; the second son Anne and his wife, Françoise Amy, and their first son Louis. The name of Hédelin is extinct at Nemours now, but the line continued at the time of Le Paulmier, being represented by Mme. la Marquise Thury Le Charron, wife of the Marquis, being a fourth-generation descendant of Catherine Paré.

Le Paulmier (p. 130) mentioned several others bearing the name of Paré, but was not able to establish any authentic connection between them and the family of Ambroise. Malgaigne (Intro., p. ccciii) wrote, "M. Villaume reported that in 1804,

'Napoleon, true appreciator of all meritorious people, gave to M. de Lasuse the mission of seeking at Laval descendants of A. Paré, whom he wished to honor, but he found none.—.'"

THE PARÉ PROPERTY

Le Paulmier provided on page 172 a schematic map of the block of houses in which Paré, his family and friends lived during the years of his active practice. The block lay between the rue des Augustins and the rue de l'Hirondelle, facing the Place St. Michel. An observer standing in the Place facing westward would have seen on the left a large building occupying about half of the block. This was the wine shop of Méry de Prime, Jeanne Mazelin's uncle. To the right, north, of this was a narrow passageway leading back into the house hidden from the street, but surrounded by an open court. This was the house Ambroise gave his niece Jeanne, and where she lived with Claude Viart, and later with François Fôrest. To the right of the passageway and extending to the rue des Augustins was the house of François Pichonnat, almost as large as that of Méry de Prime. Around the corner westward on the rue des Augustins and behind the Maison Pichonnat was another large house belonging to Charles de Paris, a grocer and Master Pastry-Cook. Next was the narrow little house Ambroise had built in 1562 for Guillaume Gueau and his wife Claude Périer, sister-in-law of Ambroise's brother Jean the Trunk-Maker. To the west of this house was a narrow alley leading back into the Paré courtyard. Across the alley was the small house of François Périer, Gueau's brother-in-law. These two men were Master-Painters and probably worked together. What stood beyond the Périer house I haven't been able to find out; probably another of the tall, narrow houses characteristic of the city in the 16th century. Behind Méry de Prime's shop, and facing the narrow rue de l'Hirondelle was the Maison de la Vache, which Ambroise acquired from his brother-in-law, Antoine Mazelin, in 1550. Here he lived with his first wife, Jeanne Mazelin, until sometime around 1562 when the demands for space required for his growing family, his shop or office, his museum and library, induced him

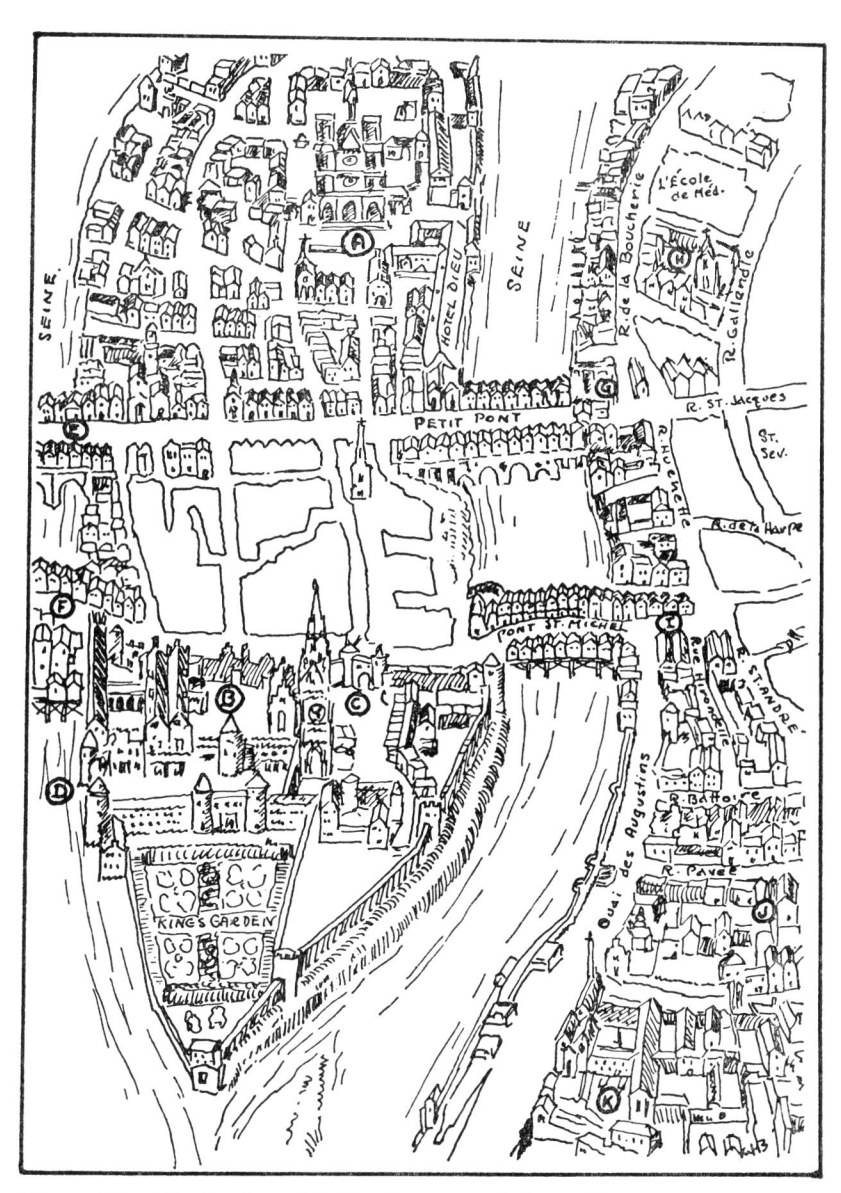

Figure 10. The Paré neighborhood in Paris (adapted from map by Truchet & Hoyou); A) Parvis Nôtre-Dame: The Cathedral is above the letter; the Hôtel-Dieu to the right; B) The Palais; C) Courtyard of the Saint-Châpelle; D) The Conciergerie; E) Pont Nôtre-Dame; F) Pont-au-Change; G) Petit-Châtelet; H) Church of St. Julien-le-Pauvre; I) Place St. Michel: Paré houses were just below the letter; J) Hôtel de Nemours; K) Convent des Grands Augustins.

to buy the somewhat larger Maison des Trois Maures (Three Moors) from the heirs of the Mestreau family. He moved into the latter house, but apparently kept the Miason de la Vache full of his appurtenances; here the widowed Jacqueline Rousselet lived after his death and here his eldest daughter Catherine returned after the death of her husband, François Rousselet, to live until her own death in 1616.

Behind the two houses facing the rue de l'Hirondelle was an open court. This had access to the outside only via the alley running between the Périer and Gueau houses, and it probably had a gate that could isolate the courtyard from the street. Le Paulmier (p. 59) said that in 1587 the entrance to Paré's "hostel" was on the rue du Quai-des-Grands-Augustins. From the courtyard, one could enter all the Paré houses, which must have been convenient, since they were all occupied by relatives by blood or by marriage.

A block south of the rue de l'Hirondelle was the rue St. André-des-Arts, on which, a block west of the Place St. Michel, was the parish church and cemetery of the same name. In 1807, a number of these old houses, especially those on the bridge, were torn down to rebuild the Quai-des-Grands-Augustins. Yet in his book of 1897, Paget said (p. 179):

> But it is the block of houses at the end of the Pont St. Michel that I love: that air of home, the sense of kinship, the quiet old-world affection of them. Take the sketch of them, adapted from Le Paulmier, and go round about it. There is the rue de La Huchette, where Jean Pare lived; the church of Saint-Andre, with a thousand memories in it, is just around the corner (it really had been gone almost a century by then). There are Ambroise's five houses, all for him and his kinfolk; at number 6, Mery de Prime, wine-seller, who also was one of the family: at number 7 lived Francois Pichonnat: at number 8, Charles de Paris, Master Pastry-Cook. Claude Viart, before he married Jeanne Pare, lived, for no less than twenty years, as Ambroise's pupil in the same house with him.

(This I have not been able to verify.)

And in a footnote he wrote:

> Eighteen years ago M. Turner believed that he had discovered Pare's house. "At the present day, in the part of the

rue de l'Hirondelle which has not yet been pulled down,[150] there is a large house which still catches your attention. It has been a great deal altered; but the door still has the shape of the doors of the Renaissance. The bit of carving over the low arch, and another carving in the wall at the back of the courtyard, have an air of antiquity. But no tradition concerning Pare is connected with it, and the present owner believes that it must have belonged to Diane de Poitiers. I am of the opinion that it is really Ambroise Pare's house.

Alas for the romanticists among us! When I made similar sentimental journeys in 1957, '59 and '61, I found the huge, traffic-congested Place St. Michel and on the Quai-des-Grands-Augustins corner is the Rotisserie Perigourdine, a famous restaurant Ambroise would have loved. Southward extends a huge block of buildings and the next corner is on the Place de St. André-des-Arts. The *Michelin Guide PARIS*, p. 45, tells us that the Place St. Michel in its present state dates from Napoleon III (1851-1873). The Place de St. André-des-Arts, according to Lansdale, p. 496, was laid out in 1810 on the site of the old church and cemetery of that name, destroyed after the Revolution. All the historic tombs it contained were destroyed and Paré's bones, mingled with the rest, were deposited in the Catacombs.[151] The present single block facing the Place St. Michel must cover at least two of the old ones of the Renaissance day. Retracing his steps, one finds an arch in the bank of buildings; this leads into the twelve-foot wide rue de l'Hirondelle. Only pedestrian traffic is possible here; one goes down a half-dozen stone steps to get to the street level. Immediately on the right is a wall with a wide-arched gateway in the center of which is carved a salamander, device of François I. Beyond the doorway is a thirty-foot courtyard with a stair leading upward. On its lintel is another salamander. This must be the house of which Turner wrote. While the house obviously is old, the state of preservation of its carvings seems too good for relics of the 16th century. From M. Jacques Wilhelm, Conservator of the Musée Carnivalet, I found that this house actually dates from the early 19th century, when the counterfeiting of architectural "trademarks" was a common practice. Now the rue de l'Hirondelle is only about fifty yards long, ending blindly at the rue Gît-le-Coeur, probably replacing the name of the rue Battoire on the old maps of the 16th century. Probably, all of Paré's property now lies under the pavement of the Place St. Michel (de Rochelle), as it did, indeed, at the times of Paget and Turner.

It is difficult to compare the city maps of the 16th century with those of today. The old ones were drawn in perspective, looking down obliquely upon the area, so the outlines of the houses encroaches upon the cross streets. These were very narrow then, so a map that shows streets running any direction except radially from the observation point grossly distort proportions. To add to the confusion here, the big new boulevards of

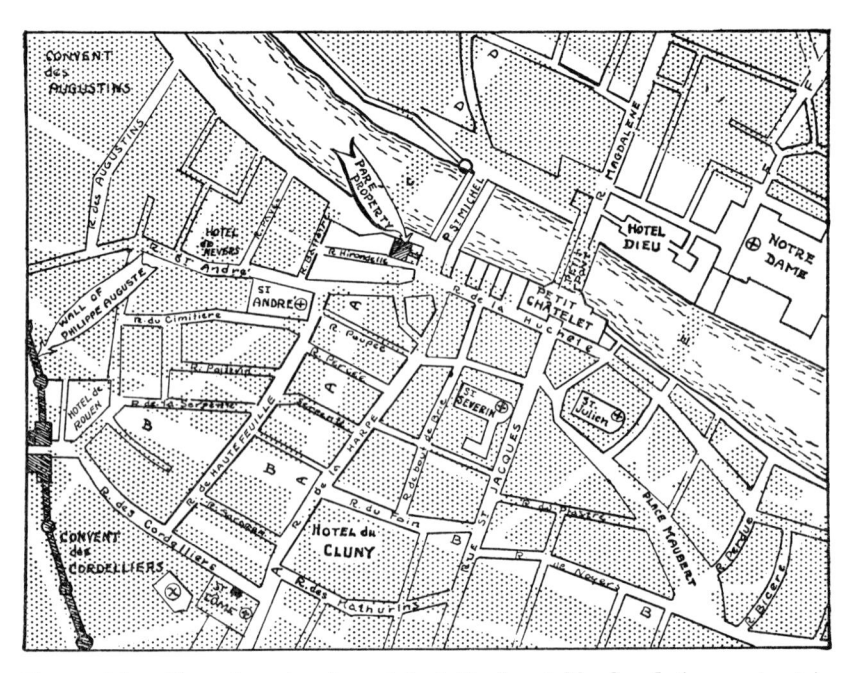

Figure 11. Alterations in the original Paré neighborhood (*approximate*), sixteenth century street plan in solid lines; present blocks stippled. A-A-A) Boulevard St. Michel; B-B-B) Boulevard St. Germain; C) Pont St. Michel; D-D) Boulevard du Palais; E) Pont-au-Double; F-F) rue d'Arcole. A portion, marked by black square, of the Church and College of St. Côme remains. Part of the Convent des Cordeliers (marked x) remains. Rue des Cordeliers is now the rue de l'Ecole de Médecine. Rue Parée is now rue Gîte-le-Coeur.

St. Michel and St. Germain were cut through this Left-Bank area in the mid-nineteenth century, leaving only traces of the major streets of Ambroise's day. Southward behind the huge fountain in the west end of the Place St. Michel, a few blocks of the narrow rue Hautefeuille extends to reach the Boulevard St. Germain in the Medical School area. This was a major traffic artery in Paré's day. The rue de la Harpe is another, only a few blocks long, running irregularly between the rue St. Severin and the intersection of the Boulevards St. Michel and St. German. The rue St. Jacques was the main Roman road from the south to the Ile-de-la-Cité; now it is overshadowed by its modern, wider neighbors.

In Paré's time, the School of Medicine was on the rue de la Boucherie, north of the Place Maubert. Later, the school was more intimately in contact with the old Hôtel-Dieu, in the neighborhood of the church of St. Julien-le-Pauvre, which for a time in the 17th century was a chapel for the hospital. The School of Medicine now occupies the sites of the old Cordelier's Convent, of which the persisting refectory is now the Musée Dupuytren. A hundred yards eastward on the rue de l'École de Medecine (old rue des Cordeliers) is a squat, octagonal-fronted building surmounted by a low, black-slate dome. Now used by the Department of Languages of the University, this building was the reconstructed church of St. Côme and later the Amphitheatre of the College of St. Côme, until the whole medical school complex was consolidated after the Revolution (Le Grand).

PARÉ'S SURGICAL INFLUENCE

As Malgaigne said in his Introduction, Paré was the first writer of his generation to fertilize the sterile surgical dust of the centuries. After the ancients, only Guy de Chauliac and Jean de Vigo had preceded him in writing classical surgical treatises. He went far beyond them. When he died, he left animated by his precepts a splendid surgical school faculty including Guillemeau, Portail, Pigray and Severin Pineau; he left the College of St. Côme on a high plane of brilliance and effectiveness. His influence fired the surgeons of Flanders, England and even Germany, where it contended with Paracelsus' doctrines and inspired them to more rapid advancement. Yet, within two generations French surgeons again were under the heavy Hippocratic yoke, and surgery in France was at as low a level as it had been when he appeared upon the scene. It remained so until Descartes "threw the light of reason into the shadows of science."

Malgaigne attributed this failure to two major factors. The first was the bitter resistance to change of that powerful, reactionary and privileged corporation, the Faculté de Médecine de Paris. The second was the prevailing moral and religious antipathy to the scientific principle. Malgaigne ascribed Paré's great success to his ardent sense of charity, to his poorly expressed but constantly demonstrated adherence to the rule of doing to others as one would wish to be done by. It was this principle the College of St. Côme forgot most quickly. This was forecast even before Paré's death in the fights of 1577. Without any sense of responsibility beyond their own gain, the surgeons continued their constant attempts to defraud the Faculté and to dominate the Barber-surgeons. They made no advances of their own, being more occupied with their own intrigues than with science. The sole means they found of maintaining the level of their College was to admit barber-surgeons whose abilities lifted them above the common level. These men were usually more able than the true surgeons, but they brought an unrecognized, so all the more fatal infection into the body of College. On admission to the College, the barber-surgeons were required to close their barber-shops and to remove such identifying ensigns from their surgeries. Remembering the insults that had been heaped upon their ancient profession by the surgeons, however, these men saw in the order only jealousy, depriving them of the opportunity to continue the trade in which they were well trained. They recognized no justice in it.

In 1610 and 1611, three able barber-surgeons, Nicholas Habicot, Jacques de Marque and Isaac d'Allemagne were admitted. Defying the imposed order, they simply added the ensign of the surgeon to their barber-poles and kept their barber-shops running. Battles raged within the College over this rebellion. Instead of maintaining their integrity and expelling the rebels, the surgeons were persuaded by the prospect of additional revenue to permit all surgeons to take on the privileges of operating barber-shops! Initially, they repeated Paré's attempt to consolidate the surgeons and the barber-surgeons into one body under the authority of the College, but again this failed. Motivated only by greed and now encouraged by the Faculté that anticipated greater abasement of their surgical rivals, in 1655 the College of St. Côme, en masse and led by their Provost, demanded and obtained their amalgamation with the Corporation of Barber-Surgeons. Only a few surgeons like Mauriceau and Dionis protested and withdrew from the association, maintaining their ancient title of Sworn-Surgeons. They cultivated the new sciences and philosophies and led the way into the 18th century rebirth of surgery. Both the Faculté and the College of St. Côme were abolished by the Revolution and were replaced by the inclusive School of Health (Le Grand).

This new breed, believing nothing impossible for the human intellect, scrapped all the ancient lore and developed a new system of surgery. The works of Paré were thrown into the dust-bins with the rest. A few men retained a curiosity about their predecessors. In 1812, the Bordeaux Society of Medicine offered a prize for an eulogy of Ambroise Paré. This was won by a Dr. Vimont; I have not found his essay. Plans were discussed for bringing out a new edition of Paré's *Oeuvres*. This was accomplished in 1840 by that prodigious worker, J. F. Malgaigne. Doe (pp. 144-152) epitomized his biography and it would serve no useful purpose to include that material here. With this stimulus, a number of studies of "le bon viellard" have appeared in English, bringing to modern readers the means of appreciating and loving this French Renaissance "Father of Modern Surgery."

The great sculptor, David of Angers,[152] modeled a life-sized statue of Paré. Funds were raised for its casting in bronze and on 29 July, 1840, it was unveiled with impressive ceremonies as it stood on a tall pediment in the Place du Novembre in Laval (Malgaigne, III, pp. xxii-xxxiii). David chose to depict Paré as a young man, standing beside a stack of five large books piled on the pedestal. An arquebus leans against them. Paré stands beside them with his head tilted forward as if in deep thought, the right hand fingering his short beard. The left arm hangs loosely from the shoulder, the fingers almost touching some writing material on the top of the stack of books. The figure looks southward across the rue de la Liberation in the general direction of the Château where Ambroise worked as a boy, and of the house where he was born.

The Paré Books

Chronology of his books appearing during his lifetime

1. 1545 *La Méthode de Traicter les Playes faictes par Hacquebutes,* etc. The first venture into print by the unknown barber-surgeon, bluntly castigating the accepted method of treating gunshot wounds (with boiling oil) and proposing a new bland dressing. His method was quickly adopted by other army surgeons, if not by the physicians. A Dutch edition appeared in 1547.
2. 1549 *Briefve Collection de l'Administration Anatomique,* etc. Based upon dissections made by himself, Thierry de Héry and Jean Colombier at l'École de Médecine, and presented as a text for barber-surgeon apprentices who, like himself, knew no Latin. A small terminal section presents the first description since the ancients of podalic version. No illustrations.
3. 1550 *Briefve Collection,* etc., consisting of a second edition of sheets left over from the first.
4. 1551 *La Manière de Traicter les Playes faictes tant par hacquebutes que par fleches,* etc. Dated 1551, but did not appear until March 1552/53. An extensive revision of the first edition, better printed, with more and better woodcuts, and better bound. Dedicated to King Henri II, at the suggestion of his Army master, the Vicount de Rohan.
5. 1552 Another edition made of sheets of the last, issued by another bookseller. Paré presented the material again in 1564 as one of his *Dix Livres de la Chirurgie,* and in all the Paris editions of his *Oeuvres* and in the Latin edition, the *Opera,* in 1582.
6. 1561 *Anatomie Universelle due Corps Humain.* A completely rewritten revision of the *Briefve Collection,* with very fair woodcuts inspired by those of Vesalius, to whom Paré acknowledged his debt. Debated anatomical details were decided by dissection with Rostaing de Binosque, and Paré's friend Caron supervised the printing and correction while Paré was away at the wars.
7. 1562 *La Méthode Curative des Playes, & Fractures de la Teste Humaine,* written at the request of the King's physician, M. Chapelain, after the fatal head wound of Henri II. A third of

the book was anatomical, taken from the *Anatomie Universelle*, published ten months earlier.

8. 1564 *Dix Livres de la Chirurgie*, etc. Includes a thorough revision of the treatise on head wounds, divided into 7 books, to which Paré added 3 new books on urology, this material taken largely from other sources. Contains his first description of the use of ligatures in amputations and abandonment of the commonly used cautery. Contains his explanation of the high mortality among those wounded in recent battles, and a description of his own leg fracture.

9. 1568 *Traité de la Peste*, etc. Written at the request of the King and the Queen-Mother, for the guidance of those treating victims of the epidemics. Of little scientific value, but is one of Paré's most systematic and best written books. Contains the controversial eulogy of antimony, deleted when rewritten for the *Oeuvres* in 1575.

10. 1574 *Cinq Livres de Chirurgie*. One of Paré's best-written books. Contains all new material; the first description of femoral neck fracture; the first systematic work since the ancients, with Paré's own added contributions, on the art of bandaging and the treatment of fractures and dislocations. It also contains Paré's "Apologie touchant les playes faictes par harquebuzades" in reply to Julien Le Paulmier's attack on his methods.

11. 1573 *Deux Livres de Chirurgie*, concerning reproduction, generation, obstetrics and monsters, all new material. This was the material responsible for the Faculté's attempt to suppress publication of his *Oeuvres* in 1575.

12. 1575 *Les Oeuvres*, etc. The collection of Paré's earlier works, expanded into a complete surgical treatise, the first since Guy de Chauliac (Malgaigne), and the first written in the Renaissance spirit of reliance upon observation and experience instead of authority. Paré was particularly proud of the illustrations, the blocks for which had cost him 1000 écus, about $5000.

13. 1575 *Response de M. Ambroise Paré, premier Chirurgien du Roi, aux calomnies d'aucuns Médecins, & Chirurgiens, touchant ses Oeuvres*. A pamphlet written to the Parlement defending his *Oeuvres* from the Faculté attack. Reprinted by Le Paulmier, 1887; not in any of Paré's own collections.

14. 1579 *Les Oeuvres*, etc., 2nd ed. Little changed from the first; the books on Animals and the Excellence of Man are new, but the material is from other sources.

15. 1580 *Traicté de la Peste*, etc., a new ed. of the 1568 *Traicté*, issued in the severe epidemic of 1580/81 as a handbook for use by barber-surgeons and others treating the victims.

16. 1582 *Discours de la Mumie,* etc., ridiculed the popular beliefs in the efficacy of mummy, unicorn's horn, etc. It was reprinted in sections in the *Oeuvres* of 1585.
17. 1582 *Opera Ambroisii Parei,* etc. Latin edition by Jacques Guillemeau, from the 2nd ed. of *Les Oeuvres,* with great liberalities by the translators. The unfortunate source of several European translations. Appearing between the 1579 2nd and the 1585 4th editions, Paré apparently considered this the 3rd edition of his *Oeuvres.*
18. 1583 *Opera* etc., a reissue of the 1582 edition with a different title page.
19. 1584 *Replique d'Ambroise Paré,* etc., *à la Response faicte contre son Discours de la Licorne.* A reply to the 1583 attack on his *Discourse on the Mummy,* defending his position admirably, logically and tolerantly.
20. 1585 *Les Oeuvres,* etc., 4th ed. The best of the original editions and the last Paré saw through the press. It contains the very important "Apologie, et Traité contenant les voyages, etc.," which throws so much light on Paré's activities and personality. It is also his final reply to the continuous attempts by the faculté to suppress and belittle his works.

This chronology has been extracted largely from Doe's splendid *Bibliography;* more complete details of the books are to be found in the text.

FOOT NOTES

Life of A. Paré

1. *Paré's age:* In his study of Paré's life, Malgaigne (Intro., p. ccxxiv) attempted to solve the problem by referring to ages noted on various portraits Ambroise had printed in his books at various times. These may be listed:

	Book	Yr. Publ.	Portrait Dated	Age Given	Birth Date Suggested
i	Anatomy Univ.	1561	Undated	45	1516
ii	Head Injuries	1561	Undated	45	1516
iii	Ten Bks. Surg.	1564	Undated	48	1516
iv	Ibid., 2nd ed.	1573	Undated	55	1518
v	Oeuvres, 1st ed.	1575	Undated	0	0
vi	Oeuvres, 2nd ed.	1579	Reprint of v.	65	1514
vii	L'Opera	1582	Undated	68	1514
viii	Mummy, etc.	1582	Undated	72	1510
ix	Oeuvres, 5th ed.	1598	1585	75	1510
x	Oeuvres, 6th ed.	1607	1584	75	1509

   This table leads to nothing but confusion, although Malgaigne noted that in his maturity, Paré favored the year 1516, and as he grew older, his birthdate became more remote.

2. *Guy XVI*, Duke de Laval until his death in 1531, married three times. His first wife, m: 1500, Catherine of Aragon, was daughter of Frederick of Aragon and of Anne de Savoy. From this marriage came four children; two died in infancy; 3) François, Count de Montfort, was killed at Biscoque in 1522; 4) Catherine de Laval married Claude, Seigneur de Rieux. Their son Réne de Rieux became Count Guy XVIII after death of his uncle Claude in 1547.

   The second marriage, 1517, was to Anne de Montmorency, sister of the Constable. Three children: 1) Claude, who became Guy XVII, married Claude de Foix, daughter of Marshal d'Odet; 2) Marguerite de Laval, married Louis V de Rohan; 3) Anne de Laval married Louis de Silli, Seigneur de la Roche-Guyon.

   The third wife, Antoinette de Dailon, daughter of Jacques de Lude, left one child, Charlotte, who married Gaspard de Coligny in 1574 (Moreri, v. 16); see version of Le Paulmier, p. 26.

3. *François I* (1494-1547) de Valois, son of Charles, Duke d'Angoulême and of Louise de Savoy, married (1514) Claude de France, daughter of Louis XII and Anne de Bretagne; became King of France in 1515. Children by Claude: 1) François the Dauphin (1518-1536), Duke de Bretagne; 2)

Henri (1519-1559), Duke d'Orlèans, King Henri II in 1547; 3) Charles (1522-1545), Duke d'Orléans in 1536, and 4) Marguerite (1523-1574) who married Emanuel-Philibert, Duke de Savoy.

4. *Nôtre-Dame Cathedral* presently probably shares equally with the Eiffel Tower as the most famous landmarks in Paris. Built and rebuilt on the site of a Gallo-Roman temple on the Ile-de-la-Cité, the present gothic structure was erected between 1163 and 1250; detail work continued for another century. It deteriorated badly and its last major restoration by Viollet-le-Duc was under Napoleon III, 1864.

5. *Hôtel-Dieu*, first charity hospital in France, established about 660 by St. Landry, 28th Bishop of Paris. Paré served as resident barber-surgeon, or "compagnon-chirurgeon" for 3 or 4 years around 1535, exact dates not recorded. It then was locted on the Ile-de-la-Cité on the south arm of the Seine between the Petit-Pont and the present Pont-au-Double, in front of Nôtre-Dame, on the plot of lawn now bearing Charlemagne's monument. Destroyed by fire in the 19th century, it was rebuilt in its present location across the island. Paré left few specific memoirs of his service there but referred proudly on several occasions to the experience he got there (Menegaux).

6. *The Grand Châtelet,* an ancient fortress on the right bank of the Seine guarding the Pont-au-Change, as early as 885 A.D. Enlarged and strengthened, it eventually became the headquarters of the Provost of Paris, with law-offices, courts and prisons. Physicians and surgeons were hired and designated "Sworn to the Châtelet" to care for prisoners and personnel. The Châtelet was rebuilt by Louis XIV but was razed in 1802, its site now marked by a Place, where a large fountain was erected commemorating Napoleon's victories.

7. *Ile-de-la-Cité:* The original town of Paris, or Lutetia, as it was called by the Romans. For several centuries, Paris was confined to this island in the Seine and was connected to the banks by two bridges, one on the north and one on the south. On the mainland, two bridgeheads served as gates and fortresses, the Grand Châtelet on the right bank and the Petit-Châtelet on the left.

8. *Nestle,* a castle and tower at the west end of the city wall of Philippe-Auguste, guarding the left bank of the Seine, at the site of the present Institute. François I gave the Little Nestle castle to Benvenuto Cellini for a workshop, as he described in his *Autobiography.* The Tour de Nestle was the scene of the alleged debaucheries of Marguerite de Bourgogne, Queen of Louis X and her sister-in-law, for which the former was strangled and the latter burned alive with her two accomplices, on the King's orders. Cardinal Mazarin (1602-1661) later left funds with which the College de Mazarin was built on the site; the left wing of the Institute and the Mint were built there following the demolition of the College (Clunn, p. 92).

9. *Henri III* (1551-1589), 4th son of Henri II and Catherine de' Médicis,

christened Edouard-Alexandre, Duke d'Anjou; elected King of Poland 1573; became King of France on death of Charles IX in 1574; married Louise de Vaudemont, no children. Early an energetic and able general, after the sojourn in Poland became a vicious, effeminate and neglectful character; was assassinated on 1 August, 1559, ending the Valois line. Was succeeded by Henri de Navarre as Henri IV.

10. *Catherine de' Médicis* (1519-1589), the Queen-Mother, daughter of Duke Lorenzo de' Médicis and of Madeleine de la Tour d'Auvergne; married Henri Duke d'Orléans, 1553, during reign of François I, who esteemed her highly. Queen of France on coronation of Henri II 1547, to whom she bore 9 children, of whom 3 became kings of France under her regency. Attempting to maintain balance of power in a divided kingdom during the Religious Wars, she attained a probably unjust reputation for dishonest intrigue and political murder.

11. *Guy de Chauliac* (c. 1300-1367), most famous medieval surgeon, born near Lyon, studied at Montpellier and Bologna. Physician of Pope Clement VI and his successors at Avignon. Wrote a classic text *Chirurgia;* French translation: *La Practique en chirurgie du Maistre Guidon de Chauliac,* Paris, 1478, was available to Paré. Latin text, *Chirurgia Magna,* Venice, 1498, was the best written surgery before Paré's (Castiglioni).

12. *Hippocrates* (460-370 B.C.), a contemporary of Socrates, Plato and Sophocles at the height of Athenian brilliance. Born on the isle of Cos into an Asclepiad (Physician-God) family, he studied medicine with his father at Athens, and traveled widely, practicing over the civilized Near-East. He disassociated medicine from theology and philosophy, crystallized the loosely knit knowledge of the Coan and Cnidian schools into a systematized science and gave physicians their highest moral inspirations. To him, the patient was the book of medical learning and his treatment the goal of the physician's existence. He instituted the case-history and his systematic writings were the basis of medical education for generations. Gradually, these became submerged and forgotten, but after rediscovery they became bible and dogma of the medical schools of the Middle Ages and the early Renaissance Universities.

13. *Galen* (131-201 A.D.), greatest Greek physician after Hippocrates. Born at Pergamus, son of an architect, went to Rome to practice in 164, was a persistent wanderer. Founder of experimental physiology, he elaborated a theoretical scheme of physiology so convincing that its errors persisted for centuries. The most voluminous of ancient writers, he left a vast and too-often misleading mass of dogma. His anatomy was developed chiefly from animal dissection because of the Roman horror of contact with the dead, and so was erroneous in many critical details when applied to the human. His contributions were enormous; it was his dogma that hindered subsequent medical progress.

13a. *Parlement:* The *Parlement* of France was developed at about the same time as the English Parliament, but the two had nothing in common. The Parlement was a court of appeals, a supreme court of the entire country, and was not a representative, legislative assembly. It was a creature of the King, developed for his convenience to take from him some of the legal load; it acted as his agent in disputes between individuals and had no control over him. Originally, it sat in Paris alone, but as bureaucracy burgeoned, Parlements independent of one another developed in all the major cities, their functions limited to their Departments, of which there are fifty-nine in modern France (Maurois).

14. *Pierre de Ronsard* (1524-1585), poet of the Renaissance, born in Vendôme. At 13, he became page for two years in the court of James V. of Scotland, then diplomatic courier for the Duke d'Orléans. Deafened by illness at 16, he retired to a life of writing. With 6 other poets including Baif, Belleau, Muret and du Bellay, a group was formed called Les Pléiades. His work so charmed Charles IX that he gave him 2 priories and 2 abbeys. He enriched the language and perfected poetic techniques. He died in his priory at Tours in 1585.

15. *Dr. Jean Fernel* (1485-1558), born at Clermont-sur-Oise, graduated at Paris, student of the classics and mathematics, then of medicine. Fascinated by astrology, he abandoned it only after years of study. He saved the life of Diane de Poitiers, winning the gratitude of Henri II, who offered him the post of Premier-Physician; deferred to M. de Bourges, taking the post of Physician-in-Ordinary. On death of de Bourges, he became Premier in 1556. Author of a 7 v. work on pathology and of a system of medicine. Went to Calais with Henri in 1558, returned to find his wife mortally ill at Fontainebleau; he died a week after her (Sherrington).

16. *Jean de Vigo* (1460-1525), born at Rapello, was brought to Rome in 1503 as his surgeon by Pope Julian II. Author of *Practica Copiosa ni Arte Chirurgica,* 9 v., Rome, 1514, went through 21 (Malgaigne) or 40 (Castiglioni) editions; translated into several languages. The work was a compilation; he added nothing important new of his own. de Vigo disappeared about 1525, place and time of death unknown (Malgaigne, Intro., clxxv).

17. *André Vésale, or Vesalius* (1514-1564), famous anatomist, son of the apothecary of Emperor Charles V, born near Brussels 31 December, 1514, studied anatomy under Sylvius in Paris (1531-1536). In 1537, he returned to Brussels, then went to Padua where he graduated in medicine the same year. Assuming the chair of anatomy the same day, he studied and taught until 1543, developing his famous *Fabrica.* After visiting Venice and Ferrara he went to Basle where his huge *de humani corporis fabrica* was published by Joannis Oporini in 1543. Immediately made famous, he returned to Brussels to practice; was Court Physician of Charles 5, 1544-1546, and of Philip II until 1564. He was very unhappy in Spain, his work stifled by the religious climate of the Court. In 1564, he appeared in Venice on his way to Jerusalem, said to have been ordered by the Inquisition in expiation for having opened a living person's chest, thinking him dead, and finding the heart beating; very improbable. He died of a fever and was buried in Zante, in Greece (Lind).

18. *St. Louis, Louis IX* (1215-1270), son of Louis VIII and Blanche of Castile; he succeeded to the throne aged 12 under his mother's regency; a very worthy king. Successful against the English in 1243, he went on a crusade to the Holy Land in 1248. Captured by the Moslems, he was freed for a huge ransom (800,000 bezants, approx. $1.8 million). He returned to France to strengthen and improve the country. In 1270, he embarked on another crusade but encamped at Tunis and died of the plague. He was canonized in 1297 by Pope Boniface VIII *(World Book Encyclopedia).*

19. *Charles IV* (King 1322-1328), known as The Good, or The Fair, the last of the Capetian kings of France.

20. *New Year:* Prior to 1563, the year in France was not uniform in length. It began variously at Xmas, on January 1, or more commonly at Easter. In 1563, Charles IX fixed the first day of January as the legal beginning of the year; the Parlement ratified the edict in 1567, but various reporters took considerably longer to adopt the rule.

21. *Charles V, Emperor* (1500-1558), grandson of Ferdinand of Aragon and of Isabella of Castile, and of Emperor Maximillan I and Mary of Burgundy. Inheriting the Spanish dominions in 1516 and the Austrian and Burgundian in 1519, he was elected Emperor of Germany and of the Holy Roman Empire the same year, defeating François I for the title. He fought François and Henri II through his entire reign over the Burgundian and Italian states, sacking Rome and capturing the Pope in 1527. Later, he persecuted the Protestants in the Netherlands and banished them from Spain. A gluttonous eater, he suffered severly from gout, which impelled his abdication in 1556 in favor of his son, Philip II of Spain.

22. *Anne de Montmorency* (1492-1567), the Constable. A very important Duke of France, descendant of the "First Christian Barons" and builder of Chantilly. Companion-at-arms of François I, Marshal of France appointed Grand Constable in 1538; he fell from François' favor in 1541, restored by Henri II, whose mentor at arms he was. A staunch Cahtolic during the Religious Wars, he was paralyzed by a spinal wound in 1557 at St. Denis. Paré treated him in his terminal illness, but he died of uremia (De Crue).

23. *Claude d'Annebault* (-1552), Baron de Retz, King's Councillor and Chamberlain, Captaine d'Evreux and Chevalier of the Order of St. Michel. He was captured with François I at Pavia, named Lieutenant-General in Normandy in 1536, Marshal of France in 1538, Governor-General of Piedmont in 1538, Ambassador to Venice in 1539, and Admiral of France in 1544; died at La Fére in 1552.

24. *Réne, Duke de Montejan in Anjou,* of Silli and of Beaupréau, Governor of Piedmont 1537, Marshal of France 1538. He married Philippes de Montespedon, no children. The Duke died in 1537 in Turin.

25. *Theriac,* misinterpreted by Johnson in the first English edition of Paré's *Oeuvres* as "treacle" or syrup, and so reprinted subsequently. In Paré's day, this was a sovereign remedy for serious wounds and diseases and

he was as credulous of its virtues as he was dubious of other nostrums. It was a complicated fermented and distilled compound including the flesh and venom of snakes. Paré listed at least three different formulas for its preparation (Malgaigne, II pp., 599-600 and, III, p. 368).

26. *Philippes de Montespedon,* only daughter of Joachim de Montespedon, Baron de Chemillé and Seigneur de Beaupréau and of Jeanne de la Haye. She married Réne, Duke de Montejan; had no children; was widowed in 1537. She married with Charles de Bourbon, Prince de la Roche-sur-Yon: 3 children. She died in her hotel, Faubourgs St. Germain, 12 April, 1578 (Le Paulmier, p. 94).

27. This may well be the first reported case of treatment of acute traumatic hemothorax (De Larouelle and Sendrail, p. 225). Most of such cases became infected and were drained subsequently as empyemas.

28. *Thierry de Héry* was born in Paris, studied at the Hôtel-Dieu with Paré and went with the French army to Rome in 1537, where he studied syphilis at the Hôspital St. Jacques Majori. On return to Paris, he studied with Drs. Jacques Houllier and Antoine Saillard. Together, he and Paré were examined and licensed as Master Barber-Surgeons, 1541, and dissected together preparing Paré's *Anatomy*. In 1544, he was with the army at Jâlons. He was appointed Lieutenant of the King's Premier Barber-Surgeon and became wealthy with a large practice. Published *La Méthode curatoire de la Maladie Vénérienne,* Paris, 1552. He died between 1552 and 1561.

29. *Dr. Jacques Houllier,* variously spelled by Paré, mentioned several times as consultant. He was called a Regent Physician of the Faculté de Médecine and praised highly; I have no other information about him.

30. *Sylvius, Dr. Jacques du Bois* (1478-1555), born at Louvilly, near Amiens. He studied anatomy under Tagault and graduated in medicine at Montpellier. In Paris, he was appointed Professor of the Faculté and became famous as an anatomist. He died 13 January, 1555, and was buried in the Cemetery for Poor Scholars.

31. See Paré *Geneaology,* p. 11, for details of Jeanne Mazelin's family relationships.

32. *Étienne de la Rivière* was a barber-surgeon of Paris who collaborated with Dr. Charles Estienne to publish the best illustrated renaissance book on *Anatomy* before Vesalius' *Fabrica*. Most of the dissections and many of the illustrations were done by Rivière. While a lawsuit held up publication, and Rivière was granted recognition, he was admitted into the College of Surgeons before the book appeared. He became Surgeon-in-Ordinary of Kings Henri II and François II and an official of the College. He helped examine Paré on his admission in 1554. An early friend of Ambroise, he witnessed his marriage to Jeanne Mazelin, was his confidant and advisor on the question of using the ligature instead of the cautery for hemostasis in amputations and treated Paré for his leg fracture in 1561. He died on 5 July, 1569.

33. *Loys Drouet,* Master Barber-Surgeon of Paris, one of Paré's early friends. He died before the publication of Paré's book on gunshot wounds in 1552.

34. *Charles Estienne* (1503-1564) was born in Paris, brother of the famous printers, François and Robert Estienne, son-in-law of the printer Simon de Colines. He graduated in medicine in 1542. A distinguished anatomist, he and de la Rivière prepared an ambitious *Anatomy* published in 1545, more than a year after the *Fabrica* appeared, due to delay caused by a lawsuit between the two collaborators. His daughter Nicole married Dr. Lièbault. In 1551, Robert Estienne fled to Geneva and Charles ran the publishing house. Arrested later himself, Charles died in prison in 1564 (Le Paulmier, p. 234).

35. *Réne, Vicount de Rohan,* Count de Poorhoët and de la Garnache, de Beauvoir-sur-Mer and of Carentan, Prince de Léon. In 1534, he married Isabelle d'Albret, daughter of Jean d'Albret and Catherine de Foix and sister of Henri d'Albret, King of Navarre. He was Paré's second Master-at-War, to whom Ambroise dedicated his book on *Anatomy* in 1549. He was killed at St. Nicholas, near Nancy 4 November, 1552 (Le Paulmier, p. 24).

36. *Charles de Cossé* (1506-1563), Count de Brissac, called "le Beau Brissac," was successively appointed Colonel of Infantry, Colonel-General of Light-Cavalry, Grand Master of Artillery, Marshal of France, then Governor of Picardy. He married Charlotte d'Esquetot by whom he had 4 children. His daughter Diane married Charles de Mansfeld, whom Paré treated after the battle of Moncontour in 1569. The great warrior died of gout 31 December, 1563 (Le Paulmier, p. 25).

37. *Heinault,* an ancient province including territory now parts of northern France and southern Belgium.

38. *Duke d'Estampes, Jean de Brosse,* son of Réne de Brosse, partisan of the Constable de Bourbon and of Jeanne, daughter of Philippe de Commines. François I had him marry his favorite, Anne de Pisseleau, for which he made him Governor of Brittany.

39. *Duke de Laval.* Le Paulmier (p. 26) identified this Duke as Guy XVI, but according to Moreri, Guy XVI died in 1531. This, then, was Guy XVII, who married Claude de Foix. They had no children. Guy XVIII was Réne de Rieux, nephew of Guy XVI.

40. *Guillaume de la Marck,* Duke de Cleves, married the 12-year-old Jeanne d'Albret in 1541, won the battle of Sittard in 1543; was captured by the Imperialists later that year, so enraging François I that he had the marriage annulled. Jeanne thus was free to marry Antoine de Bourbon in 1548.

41. *Étienne Gourmelen,* born in Brittany, graduated in medicine, Paris, 1561. Dean of the Faculté 1574-1575, appointed Professor of Surgery of the Royal College by Henri II. He led the Faculté in a series of harrassments of Paré for presuming to write in French on surgery. Paré responded in 1575, the rare tract being reprinted by Le Paulmier, p. 223. His own

Surgery, 1580, was obsolete at publication and had no second edition. He died at Melun in 1593 and is remembered only as a stimulus to the publication of Paré's *Journeys in Divers Places.*

42. *François de Lorraine and de Guise* (1519-1563), born at Bar-le-Duc, son of Claude, Count de Guise, de Lorraine and d'Aumale, Duke de Guise in 1527 and of Antoinette de Bourbon. François became a famous general and second Duke de Guise on the death of his father in 1550. He was a suitor of Jeanne d'Albret, who refused him rather than become a sister-in-law of Louise de Brézé, Diane de Poitiers' daughter, who married François' brother Claude. In 1549, François married Anne d'Este, by whom he had four famous children. He was assassinated on 18 February, 1563, near Orléans.

43. *Gaspard II de Coligny* (1516-1572), son of Gaspard I de Coligny (1470-1522) Marshal de Chatillon and of Louise de Montmorency, sister of the Constable. He became Duke de Coligny on death of his father in 1522 and Admiral of France in 1552. He married Charlotte, daughter of Guy XVI de Laval by whom he had 7 children. After her death, he married Jacqueline d'Autremonts. He became a Huguenot leader and his assassination in 1572 initiated the Massacre of St. Bartholomew's Day.

44. *Antoine de Bourbon* (1518-1562), Duke de Vendôme, oldest son of Charles Count de Vendome and of Françoise d'Alençon; brother of Condé, of Enghein, of the Cardinal de Bourbon and of Jean, Duke de Soissons. In 1548, he married Jeanne d'Albret and thereby became King of Navarre a year later. Their son Henri became Henri IV in 1598. Antoine was mortally wounded in 1562 at Rouen and was interred at the Château Gaillard.

45. *Jacques d'Albon,* Count de St. André, Marshal of France in 1547. He was King's Lieutenant at Verdun and arranged to get Paré into Metz. He was killed at the battle of Dreux in 1562.

46. *Charles* (1525-1574), Cardinal de Guise in 1547, 2nd Cardinal de Lorraine on death of his uncle Jean in 1550. He was a younger brother of François, Duke de Guise.

47. *Louis de Guise* (1527-1578) younger brother of François and of Charles Cardinal de Guise, became Cardinal de Guise in 1553.

48. *Dr. Philippe de Flexelles* graduated at Paris in 1528; according to his epitaph, Physician-in-Ordinary to Kings François I, Henri II, François II and Charles IX. At his own request, he was on the Faculté commission in its quarrel with Paré in 1559. He died in 1562 (Le Paulmier), p. 191).

49. *Dr. Louis de Bourges* (1482-1556), called Burgensis and Dr. de Gaugier, born at Blois, son of Jean Bourges, physician of the Duke d'Orléans, who was Louis' godfather. Graduated at Paris in 1506, Physician-in-Ordinary of Louis XII in 1504, of François I in 1515, and Premier-Physician in 1527, retaining this post under Henri II until his death in 1556. He assisted in liberating François I from Spain, for which he was made

Seigneur de Gaugier and de Mesland in Touraine (Le Paulmier, p. 37).
49a. *Étienne Dolet*, savant, editor and printer, was persecuted as a heretic by the Sarbonne for his Protestant writings, but was protected during her lifetime by Marguerite de Navarre. In 1546, he was tried, tortured and then hanged and his body burned with his books in the Place Maubert. In 1888, a bronze statue of him was erected to his memory at the site of his execution; the Germans melted down the figure for its bronze in 1942 (Clunn).

50. *Nicole Lambert*, Surgeon-in-Ordinary of Kings François II and Charles IX. He was among the witnesses of Paré's autopsy of Charles IX in 1574 and was godfather of Paré's short-lived son Isaac in 1559.

51. *Lansquenets*, professional mercenary soldiers, first organized in Switzerland, later from Germany and surrounding areas.

52. *Jean Philippe II*, Count Ringrave de Dauhn (1545-1569), oldest son of Philippe-François de Dauhn and of Marie-Egyptienne, Countesse d'Oettingen, married (1566) Diane de Dommartin, cousin of Christophe de Bassompierre (Le Paulmier, p. 70).

53. *Ferdinand Alvarez de Toledo*, Duke d'Alva (1508-1582), Spanish general and statesman who now is remembered outside Spain chiefly for his tyranny in the Low-Countries. He commanded several Imperial armies against the French, under Charles V and Philip II. Governor of the Netherlands in 1567, his oppression made life almost unbearable for the inhabitants. Holland and Zeeland rebelled and destroyed his fleet, causing his return to Spain.

54. Probably erroneous spelling of d'Enghein. At this time, this would be Jean de Bourbon, Duke de Soissons, whose brother François had borne the title until his death in 1546. Count Jean was killed at St. Quentin in 1557.

55. *Louis de Bourbon*, Prince de Condé, son of Charles de Vendôme, head of the House of Bourbon; brother of Antoine, King of Navarre, of François, Count d'Enghein, of Charles Cardinal de Bourbon and of Jean, Duke de Soissons. He married Eleanor de Roye, a niece of Coligny. Condé became a great Huguenot general and was killed at the battle of Jarnac in 1569.

56. *Louis de Bourbon*, Duke de Montpensier, brother of Charles, Prince de la Roche-sur-Yon.

57. *Charles de Bourbon*, Prince de la Roche-sur-Yon, Lieutenant-General of the King's armies 1557, Governor of Dauphiné 1562. Le Paulmier, p. 64, said that he was the son of Jean II and Isabelle de Beauvais, which seems unlikely, since they were a century apart in ages. I have not found his exact lineage. He married Philippes de Montespedon, widow of Réne de Montejan: three children. Paré treated him at Biarritz in 1564; he died in 1565 (Packard, p. 193).

58. *Jacques de Savoy* (1531-1585), Duke de Nemours and de Genevois, son of Philippe de Savoy and of Charlotte d'Orléans. In 1566, he married Anne d'Este, widow (1573) of François, Duke de Guise. They had

several children, one of whom, Charles, was godfather of Paré's daughter Anne, 1575.

59. *François de Seipieaux*, Seigneur and Marshal de Vielleville and de Duretal. According to Paget, p. 135, he was not Marshal at this time, getting that appointment in 1562. He died 30 November, 1571.

60. *Horace Farnese*, Duke de Castro, nephew of Pope Alexander Farnese. After the siege of Metz, he returned to Paris where he married Diane de France, the King's bastard daughter by Filipa Ducci, from the Turin days. From his honeymoon, the Duke went to the defense of Hesdin where he was killed in July 1553.

61. *Charles de Luxembourg*, Vicount de Martigues, son of François II de Luxembourg and of Charlotte de Brosse. He was married to Claude de Foix, widow of Paré's friend Guy XVII, Duke de Laval. He was mortally wounded at the defense of Hesdin where Paré treated him in 1553.

62. *François de Vendôme*, Vidame de Chartres, son of Louis de Vendôme. He won the favor of Catherine de' Médicis and the hatred of Diane de Poitiers by refusing to marry the latter's second daughter. After Henri's death, he conspired with Catherine against the Guises and the Duke forced her to send him to the Bastile. He died on the day of his release a few months later (Packard, p. 198).

64. *Pierre d'Aubert*, Surgeon-in-Ordinary of Henri II, François II and Charles IX. Le Paulmier, p. 191, reported a donation given him in 1560 in recompense for his services and for injuries inflicted upon him in 1557 before Calais by marauding soliders.

65. *Isnard Rostan de Binosque (Binosc)*, a surgeon from Provençe who began working with Paré around the time of his trip to Metz in 1552. He collaborated in the preparation of the *Anatomie Universelle*, 1561. He died in 1562.

66. *Emmanuel-Philibert*, Duke de Savoy (1528-1580), called the "Iron-Head." Born in Chambery, son of Charles III and cousin of Jacques de Savoy, Duke de Nemours. He was an able general under the Emperor at Metz and Hesdin and won the battle of St. Quentin (St. Laurence's Day) from the Constable in 1557. After the Peace of Château-Cambriesis in 1559, he married Marguerite de Valois, sister of his late adversary, Henri II. The wedding was the occasion of the tournament in which Henri was mortally wounded. Savoy retired thereafter.

67. *Guillaume du Bois*, Surgeon-in-Ordinary of Henri II. He was an official in the College of Surgeons at Paré's induction in 1554 and witnessed his autopsy of Charles IX

68. *Barnabe le Vest*, born at St. Denis, Provost of the College of Surgeons in 1554, died in 1570 (Le Paulmier, p. 43).

69. *Nicolaus Langlois*, born in Paris, Provost of the College of Surgeons, died in 1588. In 1574, he made a donation to the College resulting in a lawsuit

in which Paré figured, concerning alterations of the statutes of the College (Le Paulmier, p. 45).

70. *Jean Le Gay*, graduated in 1546, Master in Surgery, died 1548, buried at St. Severin's church (Le Paulmier, p. 48).

71. *Nicole Rasse des Neux*, born in Paris, son of a surgeon of the College of St. Côme; surgeon of Kings François II, Charles IX and Henri III; died after 1548 (Le Paulmier, p. 46).

72. *Church of St. Côme and St. Damien* was at the S.W. corner of the rues de la Harpe and des Cordeliers, at present the Blvd. St. Michel and the rue de l'École-de-Medecine. It was demolished in 1832 when the Theatre Français (Odeon) was built and the rue Racine was extended to the rue de la Harpe. In 1694, the College of St. Côme built a school on the site of the ancient College de Bourgogne, across the street, north of the church. In the next century, this fell into ruin and was replaced on the south side of the street by Gondoin's great amphitheatre in 1775. In the 19th century, a large part of this was destroyed by fire, although the low-domed part of the building still stands on the rue de l'Écol-de-Medecine and is now used by the Department of Languages of the University. The Revolution consolidated the Faculté and the College of Surgeons, and the School of Practice was built on the site of the old Cordeliers Convent, the refectory of which is now the Musée Dupuytren (Le Grand).

It will be recalled that the Corporation of Barber-Surgeons held its meetings in the church of St. Sepulcre, which was on the rue St. Denis, on the right bank of the Seine.

73. *Dr. Jean Riolan*, born at Amiens, graduated in medicine in 1548, died in 1601. Dean of the Faculté in 1548, he quarreled constantly with Paré. A generation later his son Jean, a famous anatomist, argued violently with William Harvey over the circulation of the blood.

74. *Philip II* (1527-1598), only son of Emperor Charles V and of Isabella of Portugal, succeeded to the throne of Spain 1556. Early educated as a cleric, his lifelong aim was the advancement of the Catholic Church; he strongly supported the Inquisition. He lost the Netherlands after 30 years of revolt against his tyranny, the majority of the New World holdings and Spain's place as First Power in Europe. He married: 1) Maria of Portugal; 2) Mary Tudor of England; 3) Elizabeth de Valois, and 4) Anne of Austria. The repressive atmosphere of his Court led to the ruin of Vesalius. He built the Monastery of El Escorial outside Madrid, to which he retired to die.

75. *François de Cleves* (1539-1562), Duke de Nevers, Count d'Auxerre, de Rethel and d'Eu, Seigneur d'Orval, Governor of Champagne. He married: 1) Anne de Bourbon, and 2) Jacqueline de Longwe. He commanded the French army at Laon before the battle of St. Quentin and died of an accidental pistol-shot wound of the thigh before the battle of Dreux, 1562, all within 23 years (Paget, p. 147).

76. *Antoine Portail*, born at Bearn c. 1530; came to Paris in suite of Jeanne

d'Albret; he studied and qualified as a Master Barber-Surgeon, worked with Paré at Doullens 1558. Thereafter, he married Jacqueline de Prime. Later, he was admitted to the College of Surgeons. He became Surgeon-in-Ordinary to Kings Henri II, Charles IX, Henri III, and Henri IV. The latter made him Premier-Surgeon and later elevated him to the nobility as Equyer. He and Pigray treated Henri III for his mortal wound in May 1588. Exact date of his death in unknown, but Le Paulmier, p. 376, noted that he was still Premier-Surgeon in 1608.

77. *Gabriel de Montgomery*, son of Jacques de Lorges; Captain of the Scottish Guard of Henri II. After the fatal tournament accident, he fled to England where he became a Protestant. He returned to France several times to aid the Huguenots, at Rouen and in 1573 at La Rochelle. Captured by Matignon at Domfront in 1574, he was executed in Paris (Le Paulmier, p. 50).

78. *Marie Stuart* (1542-1587), better known to us as Mary, Queen of Scots, was the daughter of James V of Scotland and of Marie, sister of François de Guise. After the age of six she was raised in the Court of Henri II, and in 1558, at the age of 16, was married to François the Dauphin. A year later, on the death of Henri, she became Queen of France. Widowed a year later, she returned to Scotland to rule as Queen of her own people. Although a Catholic, she made no attempt to impose her religion upon her predominantly Protestant country. Her marriage to her cousin Henry Stuart, Lord Darnley, brought on great religious strife and she was forced to abdicate and seek refuge in England. Elizabeth kept her a prisoner for 19 years and finally had her executed in 1587. Only in 1925 did careful re-examination of all the legal evidence finally prove her innocent of the charges for which she was beheaded. Her son became King James I of England.

79. *Nicole Lavernault (or Lavernot)* was surgeon of François I and of the Dauphin Henri and finally Premier-Surgeon of Charles IX, in which post he died in 1561, to be succeeded by Paré. He was an official of the College of Surgeons on Paré's induction in 1554.

80. *Huguenot*, the name given French Protestants, being a corruption of the German *Eidgenossen*, or Confederate, referring to the Confederated Protestant towns of Geneva, Fribourg and Berne (Maurois, p. 148).

81. *Dr. Jean Nestor*, born in Paris, graduated in medicine 1550. He apparently was alive when Paré wrote his book on *Fractures* in 1564, but in the account of 1575 he was termed "the defunct Nestor."

82. *Richard Hubert* was described in Paré's book on *Fractures* as Surgeon-in-Ordinary of M. Giles-le-Maistre, Seigneur de Bellejambe, and in 1575 as Surgeon-in-Ordinary of Charles IX. Le Paulmier said that he died in 1581.

83. *Germain Cheval*, an able Parisian surgeon, was one of the Commissioners who examined Paré on his induction into the College of Surgeons in 1554. He died in 1570.

84. *Dr. Jean Chapelain*, physician of Montpellier and of Paris in 1541; Physician-in-Ordinary of François I, Premier-Physician of Henri II and of Charles IX. Paré so esteemed him that he dedicated to him his book on *Head Injuries* in 1561. He died of the plague at the siege of St. Jean d'Angély on 5 December, 1569, in the same house where Dr. Castellan had died of the same disease a month earlier (Le Paulmier, p. 51).

85. *Laurent Colot*, also spelled Collo by Paré, came from a family of famous lithotomists. Laurent was a physician of Trainel, near Troyes. Having learned lithotomy from Marianus Sanctus, he was called to Paris in 1556 by Henri II as Surgeon-in-Ordinary and Lithotomist of the Hôtel-Dieu. The post passed to his son Laurent and his descendants. He was surgeon also to Kings François II and Charles IX.

86. *Jacques Guillemeau* (15??-1612) was born in Orléans "in 1550" (Le Paulmier, p. 75). This obviously is incorrect; he was a surgeon of François II in 1559 (Le Paulmier, p. 192). He was one of Paré's favorite pupils and lived in the Paré home for eight years, as Paré said in a poem he wrote in Guillemeau's book on *Diseases of the Eye* in 1585. Garrison called this the best Renaissance book on the subject. He served the armies and was Surgeon-in-Ordinary of Kings François II, Henri III, Henri IV, and Louis XIII. His name is not on Le Paulmier's list of surgeons of Charles IX. He published the Latin edition of Paré's *Oeuvres* in 1582, attributing the actual translation to an unnamed friend, although he himself was a classically educated surgeon. He was Provost of the College in 1595. In 1599, he saved the life of Paré's daughter Anne Simon from puerperal hemorrhage by inducing labor as he had learned from her father. He died 3 March, 1612.

87. *Dr. Pierre le Fèvre (Lefèvre)* was Physician-in-Ordinary of Kings Charles IX and Henri III and of Catherine de' Médicis. He and Paré consulted on many cases and he witnessed Paré's autopsy of Charles IX.

88. *Dr. Honore Duchastel Castellan (called Castellanus).* Physician of Montpellier in 1544, then Professor; Physician-in-Ordinary of Kings Henri II, François II, and Charles IX, and Premier-Physician of the Queen-Mother. Paré dedicated to him his book on the *Plague* in 1568. A year later, 4 November, 1569, Castellanus died of the plague at the siege of St. Jean d'Angély. His son Alexander became the King's secretary. His nephew by his sister Louise, Dr. André du Laurens, became Premier-Physician of King Henri IV (Le Paulmier, p. 63).

89. In 1895/6, *Paul Valet* had the opportunity of inspecting the old records of the churches of St. Severin and of St. André-des-Arts. In the latter, he found 2 records of Paré as godfather: 1) of 9 April, 1553, at the baptism of Genevieve Greaume, daughter of Marie du Pays, and on 21 March, 1578, when Paré and Guillaume Loquet were godfathers for Ambroise, son of Claude Viart and of Jeanne Paré.

90. *Pierre Pigray* (1531-1613), born in Paris, lived in Paré's house for several years as a pupil. He was an army surgeon and qualified as Master-

Surgeon in 1564; was appointed Surgeon-in-Ordinary by King Charles IX, Henri III and Henri IV. He and Portail were with Henri III when he was assassinated in 1588. Pigray was Dean of the College of Surgeons in 1609; he died in 1613.

91. *Jean Cointeret*, a Paris surgeon sworn to the Châtelet, died 13, May, 1592 (Le Paulmier, p. 62).

92. *Pierre Franco*, born at Turriers near Sisteron (Basses-Alpes) at the opening of the 16th century, was a celebrated surgeon practicing first in Provençe, then in Switzerland, and finally at Orange. A self-educated surgeon, he excelled at lithotomy and the surgery of hernia. He was inventor of the suprapubic approach to the bladder and prepared several skeletons for the Berne Museum. His published works of 1556 and 1561 are remarkable. The date of his death is unknown (Le Paulmier, p. 63).

93. *Dr. Nostradamus, Michel de Nostradame* (1503-1566), born in St. Rémy, grandson on his paternal side of a physician of Réne d'Anjou, King of Jerusalem and Sicily, and on his maternal side of a physician of Réne's son Jean Duke of Cambria. Educated at the University of Avignon, where he was a student-teacher of astronomy, and at Montpellier's Faculté de Médecine, he took his medical degree in 1529. He followed a peripatetic practice over Europe, spending several years at the Court of France where he was a favorite of Catherine. He retired to Salon-in-Provençe where he died in 1566. His cryptic, rhymed predictions have been reprinted several times during world crises, the last during World War II, to astound the credulous, who profess to find them pertinent to affairs of the moment.

94. *Dr. Jean de Mazille*, physician at Montpellier 1539, practiced at Beauvais. He became physician of François d'Alençon, later of François II, then Premier-Physician of Charles IX following the death of Dr. Chapelain in 1569 and Physician-in-Ordinary of Henri III. Le Paulmier, p. 191, reported stories of Catherine wanting him hanged for a favorable prognosis given during Charles' last illness, but this is discounted by his appointment by Henri III.

95. *Marie Touchet* (1549-1638), born at Orléans, was daughter of Jean Touchet, King's Councillor. She lived in the Court through Charles' lifetime and bore him two sons, one of whom died in infancy. The other became Charles d'Angoulême, whose ambitions and turbulence troubled succeeding reigns. In 1578, Marie married François de Balzzac d'Entraigues. One of their daughters, Henriette, Marquise de Verneuil, became mistress of Henri IV; the other was mistress of the Marshal de Bassompierre, by whom she had a son. Marie died in a retreat in Paris, age 89 (d'Eschevannes, p. 119).

96. *Dr. Jacques le Roy*, Physician-in-Ordinary of Henri III and Premier-Physician of Queen Louise de Lorraine, was physician of Henri IV until 1599 (Le Paulmier, p. 384).

97. *Dr. Julien Le Paulmier* (1520-1588) graduated in medicine at Caen, went to Paris in 1548, and was on the Faculté in 1556. He worked at Hôtel-Dieu for four years and for ten years under Jean Fernel, who left him his books

and manuscripts. He married Gabriel Passart, was a Huguenot, fled Paris and was recalled in 1564. He published a book on *Gunshot Wounds* in 1569. He went with Marshal de Matignon to the siege of Domfront, where Montgomery was captured. Physician of Charles IX and Henri III, he retired to Caen where he died of apoplexy. In 1887, his descendant, Stephen Le Paulmier, wrote the valuable book on Paré, from which much of the actual data for this presentation were taken.

98. *Pierre Pigray* (1531-1613), was born in Paris, lived with Paré for several years as apprentice, followed the armies, qualified as Master in Sugery 1564. He was appointed Surgeon-in-Ordinary by Kings Charles IX, Henri III, and Henri IV. He was Dean of the College of Surgeons in 1609; died 15 October, 1613.

99. *Pierre-Ernest*, Count de Mansfeld, Governor of Luxembourg, Knight of the Order of the King of Spain, married the sister of François de Bassompierre, grandfather of the Marshal (Le Paulmier, p. 70). His son Charles became godfather of Paré's son Ambroise II in 1576 (Le Paulmier, p. 93).

100. *Nicole Lambert*, Surgeon-in-Ordinary of François II and Charles IX, witnessed Paré's autopsy of Charles IX and was godfather of Isaac Paré, 1559.

101. *Henri de Guise* (1550-1588) was son of Duke François and of Anne d'Este. As Prince de Joinville, he started early following in his father's foosteps; he succeeded to his father's estate and title at 13, followed his lead in Court politics and as champion of the Catholic Church. He was wounded in the left cheek and ear by a pistol-shot in 1576 to become the second Guise "Balafré." He carried an implacable hatred for Coligny, whom he suspected of having engineered his father's assassination, finally returning the favor on the eve of St. Bartholomew's Day, 1572, touching off the notorious Massacre. He conspired with the Catholic Church and Philip II to displace Henri III. The idol of Paris, he became intolerable to the King, who had him murdered at Blois on 23 December, 1558, so he even died by treachery as his father had done. Married to Catherine de Cleves, Princesse de Porcein, he sired 14 children, 3 of whom became famous.

102. *Christophe de Bassompierre*, at 18, Colonel of 1,200 cavalry, father of Marshal de Bassompierre, married Louise le Picart de Radeval 1572 (Le Paulmier, p. 70). Marshal François de B. wrote his *Memoirs* in 1870 and described the injuries of these Colonels, his kinsmen, and their treatment by Paré.

103. *Philippe III* (1526-1595) Duke d'Arschot (written Ascot by Paré), Prince de Chimay, son of Philippe II, Duke d'Arschot, by his first wife Anne de Croy. Chevalier of the Golden Fleece, Grandée of Spain, etc., married Jeanne-Henriette, Dame de Halluyn (Le Paulmier, p. 72).

104. *Charles Philippe de Croy* (1549-1613), Marquis d'Havre (written d'Auret by Paré), was posthumous son of Philippe II, Duke d'Arschot and de Croy, by his second wife, Anne de Lorraine. He thus was half-brother of Philippe III d'Arschot. He married Diane de Dommartin, widow of the

Ringrave de Dauhn, dead at Bourgueil of his shoulder wound (Le Paulmier, p. 72).

105. *Egyptiac,* a dressing made of honey and alum, commended by Jean de Vigo.

106. *Diacalcitheos,* a plaster made of oil, litharge and vitriol, used as an astringent and detergent.

107. *Maximillian II* (1527-1576), great-grandson of Maximillian I, son of Ferdinand I, Emperor in 1564, winning against Philip II; tolerant of Protestanism, his was a peaceful reign.

108. *Dr. Simon Piètre* was born at Verade, near Meaux. He graduated in 1550 and became Professor and Dean of the Faculté in 1564. He witnessed Paré's autopsy of Charles IX in 1574. He was on the Commission with Jacquart, LeComte, Ellain, Rebours and Marescot that approved publication of the Latin *Opera* of Paré's Works in 1581. Riolan later married his daughter Anna. He died in 1584 (Le Paulmier, p. 276).

109. *Dr. Michel Vaterre,* Physician-in-Ordinary of Charles IX and Henri III, Premier-Physician of the Duke d'Alençon, was ennobled in 1573 (Le Paulmier, p. 339).

110. *Dr. Alexis Gaudin,* Physician-in-Ordinary of Charles IX and Henri III and Premier-Physician of Queen Elizabeth of Austria and of Louise de Lorraine; died c. 1579 (Le Paulmier, p. 243).

111. *Dr. Regnault Vigor,* Premier-Physician of Catherine de' Médicis, Physician-in-Ordinary of Marguerite de France, of Charles IX and of Henri III. He was sent to Nancy in 1574 to treat Claude Duchesse de Lorraine (Le Paulmier, p. 85).

112. *M. de St. Pont* witnessed Paré's autopsy on 27 July, 1574, of Mme. Roger (Malgaigne, II, p. 724; Hamby, p. 101).

113. *Dr. François Brigard,* Physician of Charles IX and Henri III, Dean of the Faculté in 1558, died 1579 (Le Paulmier, p. 339).

114. *Dr. Pierre Lafillé,* Bachelor in 1550, Dean of the Faculté in 1518/19; died 1603 (Le Paulmier, p. 276).

115. *Dr. Loys Duret* (1527-1586) graduated at Paris 1552, Physician-in-Ordinary of Charles IX and Henri III, Professor of the College de France 1568. On the marriage of Duret's daughter Catherine to Arnold de l'Isle in 1585, Henri III assisted at the church and presented the newly-weds with all the gold and silver vessels used, valued at 40,000 livres (Le Paulmier, p. 216).

116. *Jean d'Amboise,* surgeon of Charles IX and Henri III; surgeon of the Châtelet, a post he voluntarily relinquished in 1560 to Robert Gaignat (Le Paulmier, p. 192).

117. *Dr. Oliver de Violanes of Troyes,* graduated at Paris 1584.

118. *Dr. Jean Roche le Bailif* (1540-1605), a Paracelsian physician who was obliged to justify his practice before the Faculté and publish his defense in 1579. He was physician of the Duke and Duchesse de Mercoeur. Le Paulmier, p. 111, told an interesting story of his death. Feeling his end near, he called in his servants one by one and piecemeal gave them all his money and furniture. His doctors came later and told him that they found the doors open and the house empty. He replied, "Goodby, then, it is time I went also, since my baggage has gone." He died soon after, on 5 November, 1605.

119. *Loys (Louis) le Brun,* born at Paris, Surgeon-in-Ordinary of Henri III; died 1581 (Le Paulmier, p. 99).

120. *Dr. Marc Miron,* born at Tours; son of François Miron, Premier-Physician of Charles VIII; graduated 1558. He went to Poland with Henri Duke d'Anjou and became his Premier-Physician when he became King Henri III. Guillaume dedicated to him the Latin edition of Paré's *Oeuvres.* He died in 1606 (Le Paulmier, p. 84).

121. *Bernard Palissy* (1510-1589), a famous French potter who discovered the art of producing enameled pottery; also a scientist and philosopher, a pioneer in geological and chemical research, a theoretical agriculturalist and author of several art books and his *Memoirs.* His financial resources exhausted, he was rescued by the interest of Catherine de' Médicis. Arrested and imprisoned as a Huguenot in 1561, he was released and appointed Queen's-Potter, with workshops in the Tuilerie gardens. Despite his influential friends, religious persecution led to his arrest and imprisonment in the Bastile where he died in 1589 (World Bk. Encyclopedia).

122. *Claude Viart,* frequently spelled Viard by Paré, was a surgeon of Nantes who practiced near Paré in Paris. He married Paré's niece, Jeanne Paré, in 1577 and lived in a house in the Paré courtyard. The two worked together for several years. Viart died between 1582 and 1584.

123. *Charles-Emmanuel de Savoy,* Duke de Nemours (1567-1595), son of Jacques de Savoy and of Anne d'Este, was Governor of Paris during the siege of 1590. Appointed Governor of Lyonnais, Forêz and of Beaujolais, he was arrested in 1593 on order of Pierre d'Espinac, Archbishop de Lyon, and was imprisoned at Pierre-Encize, whence he escaped the next year. Unmarried, he died in 1595, reported "bleeding through the skin" (Le Paulmier, p. 94).

124. *Urbain Arbalestrier,* native of Soissons, member of the College of Surgeons, died 1585 (Le Paulmier, p. 95).

125. *Dr. Henri de Monantheuil,* born c. 1536 near Reims, graduated in medicine 1568, Professor of the Royal College of Medicine 1595, Dean of the Faculté 1578/79. During the plague epidemic of 1580, he demanded that the patients be housed elsewhere than in the Hôtel-Dieu and insisted on rigid hygiene. He wrote on mathematics and left a manuscript on Hippocrates that Guy Patin acquired. He died in 1606, leaving a daughter

who married Dr. Jerome Goulu and a son Theodore, a distinguished lawyer (Le Paulmier, p. 95).

126. *Charles de Mansfeld* (1543-1595), son of Pierre-Ernest whom Paré treated after Moncontour, and of Marie de Brédérode. He married Diane de Cossé-Brissac (Le Paulmier, p. 94).

127. *Charles de Lorraine* (1556-1605), peer, Grand Écuyer, Grand Veneur de France, Count d'Harcourt, etc., Governor of Bourbonnaise, Duke d'Elbeuf in 1581. He is not to be confused with Charles III, Duke de Lorraine, husband of Claude de Valois. d'Elbeuf was son of Réne de Lorraine 1535-1566) Marquis d'Elbeuf, brother of François Duke de Guise and of Louise de Rieux, Countess d'Harcourt. He married Marguerite Chabot (Le Paulmier, p. 94).

128. Dr. *Jean Liébault of Langres*, pupil of Duret, graduated at Paris 1561; married Nicole, daughter of Charles Estienne who wrote the *Anatomy* illustrated by de la Rivière. He wrote both medical and non-medical books. He shared the ruin of his father-in-law and retired to Dijon where he died in 1596 (Le Paulmier, p. 99).

129. Dr. *Pierre Lamer*, graduated 1572, died 1590 (Le Paulmier, p. 100).

130. Dr. *Jean Haultin*, graduated 1554, Physician-en-Quartiers (3 month service) of Henri IV. An intimate friend of Paré, apparently the real translator of the *Oeuvres* into the Latin *Opera*. With Guillemeau, he attended Paré's daughter Anne Simon in 1599 (Le Paulmier, p. 100).

131. Dr. *Germain Courtin*, graduated at Paris 1576, Professor 1578, taught surgery with distinction. He obtained an order permitting surgeons to give courses in anatomy (Le Paulmier, p. 86).

132. Dr. *Jean Martin*, graduated in Paris 1572, Physician of Henri IV, died 1609 (Le Paulmier, p. 100).

133. Dr. *Claude Rebors*, graduated in 1572 (Le Paulmier, p. 100).

134. Dr. *Giles Héron*, Dean of the Faculté 1600/03, died 1607 (Le Paulmier, p. 100).

135. Dr. *Severin Pineau*, Paris physician, Paré's friend. He published this case report in his *Opusculum physiologicum et anatomicum*, Paris, 1597. He also gave Paré a specimen for his anatomical museum, consisting of a pubic bone with a long spur projecting inward and downward from the lower end of the symphysis (Malgaigne, II, p. 666).

136. *André Malezieu*, Provost of the College of Surgeons, translated Gourmelen's *Synopsis chirurgiae* in 1571; died 1585 (Le Paulmier, p. 92).

137. Dr. *Jacques d'Amboise*, third son of Jean d'Amboise, whom he succeeded as King's surgeon. Giving up surgery, he graduated in medicine in 1594 and became Rector of the University the same year. He married Louise Desportes. He and a son died in an epidemic in 1606 (Le Paulmier, p. 385).

138. *Ismael Lambert*, son of Nicole, Sworn-Surgeon, Valet-de-Chambre and

Surgeon-in-Ordinary of Henri III and of the Cardinal de Lorraine (Le Paulmier, p. 338).

139. *Jerome de la Noue,* son of Mathurin, surgeon of Henri II. He studied medicine and surgery and became surgeon of Catherine de' Médicis and of Charles IX and Henri III, sworn to the Châtelet and Dean of the College of Surgeons. He left a surgical historical manuscript in the library of the Paris Faculté de Médecine. He died in 1628, leaving several noteworthy children (Le Paulmier, p. 116).

140. *Paracelsus, Aureolus Theophrastus Bombastus von Hohenheim* (1493-1541), the most original medical thinker of the 16th century (Garrison, p. 196). Born near Zurich, the son of a learned physician, he got his degree at Ferrara in 1515 and wandered over Europe practicing and seeking a medical doctrine credible to him. Appointed Professor Medicine at Basel in 1527, he began his course by burning in public the works of Galen and Avicenna, to emphasize returning to Hippocrates and progressing on his own experience. He was put out of Basel within a year. He encouraged the development of chemistry and pharmacology, but got sadly muddled in astrology, alchemy and the occult. He died of injuries sustained in a Salzburg tavern brawl (tradition).

141. *Christophe Jouvenal des Ursins,* oldest of six children of François Jouvenal des Ursins and of Anne l'Orfèvre, dame d'Armenonville. In 1557, he married Madeleine de Luxembourg and died in 1588 (Le Paulmier, p. 105). His injury in 1580 was the stimulus for Paré's *Discourse on the Mummy and the Unicorn.*

142. *Rodolphe Le Fort of Senlis,* Provost of the College of Surgeons, who actively defended the rights of surgeons. He died in 1606 (Le Paulmier, p. 105).

143. *Oxycrate,* a mixture chiefly of vinegar and saffron.

144. *Étienne Delaulne,* French designer and engraver, born at Orléans 1519, died in Paris 1583; lived in Augsbourg and Strasbourg. He engraved a considerable number of pieces remarkable for their precision and fineness of design. He made the Paré portrait a year before his death (Le Paulmier, p. 14).

145. *Alexandre Vallée,* designer and engraver with acid and drypoint, born at Bar-le-Duc around 1558, died in the 17th century; especially active 1583-1610 (Le Paulmier, p. 14).

146. *François de Balsac d'Entraigues,* oldest son of Guillaume de B-, who was Lieutenant of a company of Guise's soldiers in Metz, 1552. Guillaume became Seigneur de Marcousies, de Nozay and of la Ville-du-Bois in 1545. He gave Nozay and Ville-du-Bois as dowry to his daughter Louise when she married Jacques Baron de Clair. On his death in 1554, Guillaume left only Marcousis to François, who repurchased Ville-du-Bois in 1580. In 1579, he married Marie Touchet (Risch).

147. *Archbishop de Lyon* at this time was Pierre d'Espinac, son of Pierre

d'Espinac, King's Lieutenant in Burgundy and Lyonnaise. He was Curé, then Dean of the Church of Lyon, Archbishop in 1574, succeeding his uncle Antoine d'Albon. He wanted to be a Cardinal; unable to attain this, he joined the Guise party, the League. Arrested with the Cardinal de Lorraine at Blois, his nephew Edmund de Malain secured his release. He died in 1599 (Le Paulmier, p. 118).

148. *Jacques Marchant*, Paris surgeon, son of Paris Master Barber-Surgeon Guillaume Marchant and of Marguerite Rousseau. In 1598, he married Marguerite, daughter of Jacques Guillemeau and of Marguerite Malartin (Le Paulmier, p. 337).

149. *Turner* located the Château de Paley in the Canton de Lorrez-de-Bocage (Seine-et-Marne), 12-15 Km from Nemours.

150. In *Turner's* 1 January report, this sentence has another clause at this point, ". . . at the base of the stair and the arcades that separate it from the Place St. Michel . . ." This indicates that at the time of his observation the condition of the street and of the house he mentions were essentially the same as at present. On p. 197 of his *Études Historiques* he said, "I was wrong in my first report when I supposed that the house in the rue de l'Hirondelle immediately at the base of the stairs on the right was actually Paré's. This is the house given by François I to the Duchesse d'Étampes." Le Paulmier, p. 26, said "It was for (her) that around 1530 the King had restored the Palais d'Amour, of which some vestiges still can be seen at Nos. 20 and 22 in the rue de l'Hirondelle." This is the house of which Turner wrote, but evidence from the Musée Carnivalet indicates that this house was built early in the 19th century.

151. *The Catacombs* is an underground depository in Paris for the remains of some five million humans. Walled Paris had insufficient cemetery space and, in times of epidemics, the land of the small churchyards and especially the Cimetiere des Innocents was reused too frequently. Ultimately, the ground level of St. Innocents stood 8 feet higher that the streets. The surrounding area became crowded with markets for food and other items, producing a dangerous hygienic condition.

Concurrently, the quarries around St. Genevieve were worked so deeply and so undercut the surroundings that by 1775 the land began to cave in seriously. Immense supporting pillars were built in the quarries, providing 150 acres of galleries connected by 1,400 meters of underground passages having 70 or more exits. The cemeteries were emptied into the quarries, the Catacombs being consecrated in 1786. The first victims of the Revolution were interred there (Clunn, p. 204).

152. *Jean Pierre David d'Angers* (1788-1856), a pupil of Canova who turned from classicism to realism. His most famous sculptures are the Condé Memorial in the Cours d'Honneur at Versailles and the Pantheon reliefs (1834). He was a member of the Institute and of the Academies of Rome, Berlin, London and New York. A special museum at Angers is devoted to his works. (Jouin, H., *David d'Angers*, Paris, 1878).

References

1. Batiffol, Louis: *The Century of the Renaissance*, London, Wm. Heinemann, Ltd., 1916.
2. Bégin, Emilé: Ambroise Paré. *Gaz. Hebd. de Med. et de Chir.*, 15:629-635, 645-653, 725-730, 1878; 16:1-7, 1879.
3. Castiglioni, A.: *A History of Medicine*, New York, Knopf, 1941.
4. Cellini, Benvenuto, *The Life of Benvenuto Cellini*, 3rd ed., newly translated into English by John Addington Symonds, London, John C. Nimmo, 1889.
5. Chaussade, A.: Ambroise Paré et Charles IX: Paré Premier Chirurgien, Le Grand Tour de France, etc. *Rev. Historique*, 156:294-323, 1927.
6. Chauvelot, R.: *Les Sources d'Ambroise Paré*: Anatomie, *La Presse med.*, 63:147-148, Feb. 2, 1955. Introduction à la chirurgie, *Ibid.*, 63:1717-1719, Dec. 10, 1955. La Manière de extraire les enfans tant mors que vivans, *Ibid.*, 66:1191-1201, and 1285-1286, 1958.
7. Chevalier, A.: *L'Hôtel-Dieu de Paris et les Soeurs Augustins, 650 à 1810*, Paris, H. Champion, 1901.
8. Clunn, H. P.:*The Face of Paris*, London, Spring Books, n.d.
9. Cushing, H.: *A Bio-Bibliography of Andreas Vesalius*, New York, Schumann, 1943.
10. De Crue, F.: *Anne de Montmorency, Grand Maître et Connétable de France*, Paris, 1885.
11. De Laruelle, L., and Sendrail, M.: *Textes Choisis de Ambroise Paré*, Paris, Soc. les Belles Lettres, 1953.
12. Doe, Janet: *A Bibliography of the Works of Ambroise Paré; Premier Chirurgien et Conseiller du Roy*, Chicago, Univ. Chicago Press, 1937.
13. D'Orliac, J.: *François I, Prince of the Renaissance*, Philadelphia, Lippincott, 1932.
14. Elliott, James: *Old Court Life in France*, New York, Putnams, 1893.
15. d'Eschevannes, C.: *La Vie d'Ambroise Paré, Père de la Chirurgie*, Paris, Libraire Gallimard, 1930.
16. Garrison, F. H.: *An Introduction to the History of Medicine*, Philadelphia, W. B. Saunders Co., 1924.
17. Guizot, M.: *A Popular History of France, from the Earliest Times* (Translated by Robert Black) v. IV, Boston, Estes & Lauriat, n.d.
18. Haberling, W.: Die Bildnesse der Ambroise Paré, *Sudhoff's Arch. f. Gesch. der Med. u.d. Naturwsnchft*, 14:106-109, 1922/23.

REFERENCES

19. Hamby, W. B.: *The Case Reports and Autopsy Records of Ambroise Paré*, Springfield, Ill., Thomas, 1960.
20. Hoefer: *Nouvelle Biographie Universelle*, Paris, Fremin Didot Freres, 1853.
21. Johnson, Th.: *The Works of that Famous Chirurgion Ambroise Parey, Translated out of the Latin and Compared with the French*, London, E:C, 1665.
22. Jouan, Abel: *Recueil et Discours du voyage du Roy Charles IX*, etc. Paris, 1566.
23. Kellett, C. C.: *Perino del Vaga et les Illustrations pour l'Anatomie d'Estienne*, Aesculape, Paris, April, 1955. A Note on Rosso and the Illustrations to Charles Estienne's "De Dissectione," *J. Hist Med.*, XII:325-337, 1957. *Two Anatomies*, Lecture Univ. of Durham, May 8, 1958.
24. Kelly, W. K.: *The Heptameron of Margaret, Queen of Navarre*, London, n.d.
25. Keynes, G.: *The Apologie and Treatise of Ambroise Paré*, etc., Chicago, Univ. of Chicago Press, 1952.
26. Lansdale, M. H.: *Paris, Its Sites, Monuments and History*, Philadelphia, Henry T. Coates Co., 1899.
27. Le Grand, Noe: *Les Collections Artistiques de la Faculté de Médecine de Paris*, Paris, Masson et Cie., 1911.
28. Le Gras, J.: *Tour de France de Charles IX*, Paris, Les Oeuvres Libres, 123, 1931.
29. Le Paulmier, Stephen: *Ambroise Paré, d'après de Nouveaux Documents*, etc., Paris, Perrin et Cie., 1887.
30. Lind, L. R.: *The Epitome of Andreas Vesalius*, New York, Macmillan, 1949.
31. Malgaigne, J. F.: *Oeuvres Complètes d'Ambroise Paré*, Paris, J. B. Bailliere, 1840.
32. Maurois, André: (Binsse Transl.) *A History of France*, New York, Grove Press, 1948.
33. Menegaux, G.: L'Hôtel-Dieu de Paris et ses Chirurgiens, *Presse Med.*, 64:2225-2229, 1956.
34. Michelet, L.: *La Vie d'Ambroise Paré (Chirurgien du Roy, Écrevain)*, Paris, Libraire le François, 1930.
35. Montagu, M. F. A.: Vesalius and the Galenists, *Scientific Monthly*, 230-239, April, 1955.
36. Moréri, Louis: *Le Grand Dictionnaire Historique*, v. 16, Paris, 1759.
37. Packard, F. P.: *Life and Times of Ambroise Paré*, New York, Paul C. Hoeber, 1926.
38. Paget, Stephen: *Ambroise Paré and His Times, 1510-1590*, New York & London, G. P. Putnam's Sons, 1897.

39. Paré, Ambroise: *Ambroise Paré, Voyages et Apologie,* Paris, La Renaissance 2, Libraire Gallimard, 1928.
40. Power, d'Arcy: Archeaologica Medica: The Iconography of Ambroise Paré, *British M. J.,* 2:965, Nov. 23, 1929.
41. Risch-Leon: *La Masion des Champs du Chirurgien Ambroise Paré à la Ville-du-Bois (Seine-et-Oise),* Arpaijon, 31, 1938.
42. Rochelle, Marquis de: *Promenades dans toutes des Rues de Paris, Par Arrondissement,* VI Arrond. Paris, Libraire Hachette, 1910.
43. Roeder, R.: *Catherine de' Médici and the Lost Revolution,* New York, Viking Press, 1937.
44. Rousselet, A.: *Notes sur l'Ancien Hôtel-Dieu de Paris, relatives à la Lutte des Administrateurs laïques contre le pouvoir spirituel,* etc., Paris, E. Lecrosnier & Babé, 1888.
45. Sedgwick, H. D.: *The House of Guise,* Indianapolis & New York, Bobbs-Merrill Co., 1938.
46. Sherrington, Sir Charles: *The Endeavor of Jean Fernel,* Cambridge, The University Press, 1946.
47. Singer, D. W.: *Selections from the Works of Ambroise Paré,* etc., London, John Bale, Sons & Daniellson, Ltd., 1924.
48. Truchet, A., et Hoyau, G.: *Plan de Paris, sous le Regne de Henri II,* Paris A Taride (Ed. I, 1877), 1908.
49. Turner, E.: *Études Historiques,* Paris, 1878.
50. Valet, Paul: *Ambroise Paré,* 1) *son Mariage à St. Severin,* 2) *Marrain à Saint-André-des-Arcs,* Bull. de la Moulagne Ste. Genevieve et des Abords, Paris T, 194-207, 1895/6.
51. Wickersheimer, C. A.: *La Médecine et les Médecines en France à l'époque de la Renaissance,* Paris, A. Maloine, 1906.
52. Wiley, W. L.: *The Gentleman of Renaissance France,* Cambridge, Harvard University Press, 1954.
53. Williams, H. N.: *Henri II, His Life and Times,* New York, Chas. Scribner's Sons, 1910.
54. *World Book Encyclopedia,* Chicago, Quarrie Corp., 1945.
55. Young, G. F.: *The Medici,* New York, The Modern Library, 1933.

Index

* indicates a surgeon or Barber-Surgeon
Italic numbers indicate Footnote reference

A

Abbeville, France: 63, 80, 85
Abdication, Emperor Charles V: xiv, 89
Abscess, neck: 121
Accusation
  false quotation: 154
  lying: 151
  plagiarism: 48, 52, 133, 182
  poisoning: 96, 162
  regicide: 96
Adder bite: 127
Admiral Coligny: 114, 143, 217
Age of A.P.: 101, *210*
Agincourt, France: 63
Aix-en-Provence, France: 118
d'Albon, Jacques, Count de St. André: 52, 60, 67, *217*
d'Albret, Jeanne: 48
d'Alençon, Duke (Herculé de Valois): 106
d'Allemagne, Isaac*: 204
d'Alva, Duke: 62, 71, 93, *218*
Amalgamation, Surgeons and Barber-Surgeons: 205
Ambi: 151
Amboise, Conspiracy of: xv
  edict of: 109
  Peace of: xvi, 109
d'Amboise, Dr. Jacques: 166, *227*
  Jean*: 148, 167, *225*
America, discovery of: 17
Amputation
  elbow joint: 34
  extremity: 35
  fingers: 143

hemostasis
  cautery: 62, 78, 170
  ligature: 62, 113, 130, 178
  painful leg: 183
Amy, Françoise: 197
Anatomie Universelle du corps humain (Paré): xv, 97, 101, 207
Anatomy
  Estienne de la Rivère: 41, 48, 51
  Paré: xiv, 39, 53, 55, 97
  Vassé: 54
  Vesalius: 48
Anatomy (*Briefve Collection*, etc.): xiv, 39, 53, 55, 97, 207
Angers, France: 13, 27
d'Angers, David: 205, *229*
Angoulême: 123
d'Anguien, M.: 67, *218*
Animals
  bites: 141
  book of: 168
d'Anjou, Duke
  François de Valois (Monseigneur): xvii, 114, 134
  Henri de Valois: 148, 173, 195
Ankle fracture (A.P.): xv, 113
d'Annebault, Claude: 27, 37, 42, 113, *214*
Antidote: 106, 128, 155
Antimony: 133, 150, 155
Antoine, Cardinal DuPrat: 24, 40
Antwerp, Belgium: 139
d'Anville, Marshall: 68
Apologie et Traite . . . . . (A.P.): xvii, 28, 42, 46, 62, 171, 185, 209
Apothecary: 67, 120, 129, 145
Appliances, orthopedic: 59, 109

233

Appointments, Royal, A.P.
  Surgeon-in-ordinary
    Henri II: xiv, 64
    François II: xv, 94
    Charles IX: xv
  Premier-Surgeon & Valet-de-Chambre
    Charles IX: xv, 103, 149
    Henri III: xvii, 149, 190
  Kings Councillor: xvii, 149
Apprentice, barber-surgeons, 21
A.P., 14
  of A.P., 42
Arabic Manuscripts, translations: 16
l'Arbalestrier, Urbain*: 162, 167, *226*
Archbishop of Lyon: 191, 193, *228*
Archer of Meudon, operation: 147
Architect: 152
Arles, France: 118, 119
Armenonville, France: 171
Arnoullet, donation: 94
Armada, Spanish: xviii
Arteriotomy, temporal: 122
Artificial limbs: 59, 62
d'Ascot (d'Arschot), Duke: 135, *224*
Assassination
  Cardinal de Lorraine: xviii, 190
  Coligny: xvi, 143
  François de Guise: xv, 109
  Henri III: xviii, 192
  Henri de Guise: xviii, 190
Astrology: 19, 118, 119, 170, 203, *223*
Aubert, Pierre*: 69, *219*
d'Aubignac, Abbaye: 197
Aufimon, France: 85
des Augustins, rue: 198
d'Aumale, Duke (Louis de Guise): 52, 191, *217*
d'Auret (d'Havre), Marquis: 135, *224*
Autopsy
  Charles IX: xvi, 148
  Chest, gunshot, M. de Martigues: 83
  dysentery: 92
  executed woman: 166
  François II: xv
  heart wound: 33
  Henri II: xv
  Henri III: 192
  hydatid mole: 150
  poisoned thief: 129
  skull fracture: 79
  traumatic thoracic hemorrhage: 47
Auvergne, France: 128
Auxerre, France: 130
Avesnes, France: 45
Avigliana (Château de Villane): 29
Avignon, France: 17, 118

B

de Bailif, Dr. Jean Roche: 151, *226*
"Balafre" (scar-face): 51, *224*
Balm
  eye: 177
  gunshot wounds: 32
Bandaging: 141
Barber-surgeons
  apprenticeship: 21
  corporation of: 21, 204
  licensure: 21, 40
  origin of: 21
  Premier: 23, 131
Barge travel: 120
Bar-le-Duc, France: 114, 115
de Bassompierre, M. Christophe: 135, *224*
Bastille: 16
Battle of
  Dreux: xv, 108
  Moncontour: xvi, 134
  Pass of Suza: 4, 29
  Pavia: 24
  St. Denis: xvi, 131
  St. Quentin: xiv, 89
Baugé, France: 125
M. de: 68, 85
Bayonne, France: xvi
  Conference of: 121, 130
le Beau, Mathurin*: 177, 181
Beaumont, Chateau: 138
Beaupréau: 124
  Duchesse de (Phillipes de Montespedon): 163, 164, *215*
de Beauregard, Philippe: 141
Beauvais: 183
de Beauvois, Josse*: 167
Beggars: 13, 53, 82, 100
Bégin, Dr. Émile: 11, 49, 76, 163

INDEX

Bjart, Armande: 58
Belgium, Paré visit: xvi, 136-139
Bequest
  Amy: 197
  Bertrand Paré: 55
  Gaultier: 126
  Gueau: 101
  Jeanne Paré: 147
  Langlois: 162
  Viarts: 164
  Will (A.P.): 189
Bezoar: xvi, 128, 154
Biarritz, France: xvi, 122
Bible, first French printing: 149
Bibliography of A.P. (Doe): 209
Bibliothèque Nationale: 111, 165
Bidache, France: 123
de Bieux, Antoine*: 149
de Binosc, Rostan (Rostaing)*: 76, 90, 97, 106, *219*
de Biron, Marshal: 68, 176, 192
Birth, A.P.: 10, 12
Bladder stone, first operation (Tradition): 146
Bleeding (Phlebotomy): 99, 117, 127
Blois, Château: xviii, 127, 190
Blood loss at amputation: 178
Blood supply, mammary: 167
de Bois-Dauphine, M.: 91
du Bois, Guillaume: 87, 134, 148, *219*
du Bois, Jacques (Sylvius): xiii, xiv, 24, 39, 49, 54, 89, *215*
Bone-setter: 115
Bonnivet, M.: 68
Bons-Hommes, village: 98
Books, A. P.: 207-209
de Bordaille, M.: 68
Bordeaux, France: 120
  Society of Medicine: 205
de Bordes, M.: 108
la Boucherie
  church: 8
  rue de: 203
de Bouchet, M.: 84
de Bouillon, Duke: 77, 79
Boulevards
  St. Germain: 203
  St. Michel: 203
Boullaie

  Marie: 145, 165
  Robert: 146
Boulogne, France: xiii, 45, 50, 55, 63
de Bouluet, Baron: 176
de Bourbon
  Antoine
    Duke de Vendôme: 52, 63, 64
    King of Navarre: xv, 90, 94, 98, *217*
  Charles, Cardinal: 105, 113, 190, 191, *218*
  Charles, Prince de la Roche-sur-yon: 67, 94, 105, 114, 122, *218*
  Henri, Duke de Vendôme: xv, 114, 142, 144, 148, 192
  King Henri IV: xv, 192, 194
  Jean, Duke d'Enghein: 67, *218*
  Louis, Prince de Condé: xv, xvi, 67, 90, 94, 104, 108, 109, 114, 132, *218*
  Duke de Montpensier: 67, 114, 218
de Bourdillon, Marshal: 90, 114
Bourges, France: xv, 104, 127, 197
  Dr. Louis de: 53, *217*
Bourg-Hersent, France: 10
Bourgueil, France: 125, 134
Bouteroue, Francois: 146
Bouvot, Madelain: 197
Brain injury: 44, 106
de Brandenberg, Marquis, 74
Brest, France: 46
Bridge, St. Michel: 57, 163, 193
Briefve Collection, etc. (anatomy), A.P.: xiv, 39, 53, 55, 97, 207
Brigard, Dr. François: 148, 225
de Briou, Hilaire, Apothecary: 145
de Brissac, Count, Charles de Cossé: 43, 216
Brittany
  campaign: 46-47
  dance: 47
Brouge, France: 124
le Brun, Loys*: 157, *226*
Brussels, Belgium: 139
Bubo: 117
Buon, Gabriel, Publisher: 149, 156, 166, 168, 170, 179, 184, 190
Burgundy
  Duke, Charles-The-Bold: 27

Governor, Gaspard de Saulx: 116
Burning
  at stake: 188
  Hôtel-Dieu: 24
Burns: 33

C

Cabrol, Bartholomey°: 119, 167
Caesarian section: 173
Calais: xv, 77, 91
Calculi
  salivary duct: 122
  urinary bladder: 146
Calendar: 102, 117, 141, 214
le Camus, Jean: 164, 188
Canappe, Dr. Jean: 53, 54
Canche, river: 78
Cappel, Dr.: 184
Capture
  A.P. at Hesdin: xiv, 81
  Constable Montmorency: 89, 108
  François de Montmorency: 77
Carbuncles: 122
Carcassonne, France: xvi, 120, 132
Cardinal
  de Bourbon, Charles: 105, 113, 190, 191, 218
  de Guise
    Charles: 52, 94, 114, 190, 217
    Louis: 217
  de Lorraine, Charles: 52, 94, 114, 190, 217
  de Richelieu: 197
Carnivalet, Musée: 201
Carounge, M: 68
Cartier, Jacques: xiii
Castellan, Dr. Honore Duchastel: xvi, 106, 114, 119, 124, 127, 133, 222
de Castelpers, Mme.: 127
Catacombs: 201, 229
Catherine de'Médicis, Queen-Mother: ix, xiii, xv, 16, 52, 77, 104, 118, 152, 191, 212
Catholic League: xvii, 191
Catholicism, Paré: 107
Cautery
  for hemostasis: 62, 78, 170
  potential: 121, 125
Cavellat, Guillaume, Publisher: 53
Cemetery
  St. André-des-Arts: 200
  St. Innocents: 229
Ceremony, Royal, medical: 103
Chailot Palace: 98
Champigny, France: 53
Chapelain, Dr. Jean: xvi, 93, 101, 106, 114, 118, 119, 124, 127, 222
la Chapelle, M. de: 68
Châpelle St. Louis (Sainte Chapelle): 103
Charbonnel, Jean°: 178, 183
Charlemagne: 24
Charles IV (le-Bon): 25, 214
Charles V (Spain, The Emperor): xiii, 26, 66-78, 89, 214
Charles IX: xv, xvi, 44, 97, 100, 103, 111-130, 140, 148, 192
Charles de Paris: 101, 198
Charles, Pierre: 169
Charles-The-Bold (l'Hardi): 27
de Charles, Vidame (Francois de Vendôme): 68, 219
Charron, Marquise Thury Le: 197
Chastel, Captain: 60
Château d'Auret: 136
Château, Beaumont: 138
Châteaubriant: 125
Château-Cambriesis, Peace of: 93
Château de Monceaux: 130, 131
Château-de-Paley: 149, 185, 229
Château de Villane (Avigliana): 29
Château-le-Comte: xvi, 62, 63
Châtelet, The Grand: 94, 96, 101, 147, 163, 188, 211
Châtillons: 109
de Châtillon, Gaspard, Duke (Coligny): xvi, 51, 59, 104, 108, 109, 114, 143, 217
de Chauliac, Guy: 17, 21, 119, 203, 212
Chaussade, A: 111
Chauvelot, R: 54
Chemical apparatus: 141
Chenonceaux, France: 127
Chest, gunshot wound: 35, 80
Cheval, Germain°: 88, 100, 221

INDEX

Cheval, Pierre°: 167
Children, Ambroise Paré:
  1. Francois: xiii, 48, 49
  2. Isaac: 95
  3. Catherine (I): xv, xvii, 96, 172, 173
  4. Anne: xvii, 161, 174, 189
  5. Ambroise (II): xvii, 162, 163
  6. Marie: xvii, 164
  7. Jacqueline: xvii, 169
  8. Catherine (II): xvii, 172, 197
  9. Ambroise (III): xvii, xviii, 182
Chirurgicae artis, ex Hippocrates, etc., Gourmelen: 170
Chirurgiens-juré (Sworn-Surgeons): 22
Choisel, Marguerite: 41
Chronique scandaleuse: 146
Chronology of A.P.: xiii
Church
  Mathurins: 88
  Nôtre-Dame: 14, 24, *211*
  St. André-des-Arts: 41, 95, 96, 106, 145, 161, 163, 164, 169, 172, 182, 194, 200
    registers of: 165
  St. Côme et St. Damien: 203, *220*
  St. Germain l'Auxerrois: 143
  St. Innocents: 134
  St. Jacques-de-la-Boucherie: 88
  St. Jean-Baptiste: 197
  St. Julien-le-Pauvre: 203
  St. Martin of the Fields: 178
  St. Sepulcre: 21, 40
  St. Severin: 146
Cinq livres de chirurgie (A.P.): xvi, 134, 140, 141, 208
Citröen factory: 58
City map (Paris): 199, 202
Civil war: 96, 131
Clement, Jacques: xviii, 192
Clement VII, Pope: 154
Cléret, Étienne: 40, 41, 96
Clermont (Clermont-Ferrand), France: xvi, 128
de Cleves, Duke (Guillaume de la Marck): 48, *216*
Clunn, H. P.: *229*
Cointeret, Jean°: 108, 148, 167, 172, 177, 178, *223*

de Coligny, Gaspard II, Duke: xv, xvi, 51, 59, 104, 108, 109, 114, 143, *217*
de Colines, Simon, Publisher: 48, 51
College of Surgeons: xiv, 23, 44, 87, 88, 153, 162, 174, 203, 205
Collot, Germain°: 146
Collot, Philippe°: 167
Colombier, Jean°: 51
Colonization of Florida: xvi
Colot, Laurent°: 103, 113, *222*
Columbus, Christopher: 17
Commission of Eight: 24
Committee, Faculté: 165
  of Sixteen: 193
Comperat, B°: 151, 187
de Condé, Duke (Louis de Bourbon): xvi, 67, 90, 94, 104, 108, 109, 114, 132, 140, *218*
  Henri: xv, 114, 142, 144, 148, 192, 194
Conference of Baylogne: 121, 130
Confraternity of St. Côme: 22, 23, 88, 131
Conspiracy of Amboise: xv
The Constable, Anne de Montmorency: 13, 27, 52, 59, 86, 89, 94, 95, 108, 112, 113, 118, 124, 132, 134, *214*
Consultations: 105, 120, 137, 147, 171, 178
Contract, Marriage
  A. Paré—Jean Mazelin: 41
  A. Paré—Jacquelin Rousselet: 145
  Jeanne Paré—Claude Viart: 163
  Jeanne Paré—François Fôrest: 190
Convent des Cordeliers: 203
Convulsions, post-traumatic: 35, 45
Copper Engraving, portrait: 179
Cordeliers Convent: 203
Coronation
  Catherine de' Médicis: 52
  Charles II, xv, 100
  Henri II: xiv, 52
  Henri III: xvii
Corporation of Barber-Surgeons: 21, 40, 205
Cortez, Conquest of Mexico: xiii
de Cossé, Charles, Count de Brissac: 43, *216*

Côte-d'Or: 116
Council of War: 71, 81
Court duties: 87
Court tour: xvi, 111-130
Coupé, Jerome: 167
Courtin, Dr. Germain: 165, 183, 227
Cousin, Jean (Artist): 101, 113
Cracow, Poland: 148
Cranial defect, prosthesis: 36
Craniopagus: 140
Crécy, battlefield: 63
Credulity, A.P.: 119
Criminal activity during plague: 116
Crinel, Solin*: 176
Crow's beak forceps: 178
Crushing injury: 177
de Culan, Baron: 81
Cushing, Dr. Harvey: 54, 84

D

Daigue, M. (Apothecary): 67
Dalechamps, M*: 116
Damvilliers, France: xiv, 61, 62, 113
Dates, confusion re.: 102, 117, 141, 214
Dativo, wrestler: 47
Daubray, M., Merchant: 169
David d'Angers (Artist): 205, 229
DeCrue, F.: 214
Decubitus ulcer: 136
Dedications, Paré books: 49, 53, 98, 101, 113, 133, 141, 142, 157, 170, 174, 179
Defense of his writings: 142, 153, 154, 182, 183, 209
De Laruelle, L. and Sendrail, M.: 215
Delaulne, Étienne (Engraver): 185, 228
Delivery (obstetrics): 141
De Nets, M. (Attorney): 188
Dentistry: 141
Deposition, legal: 95
Derision of College of Surgeons: 88
Descartes, René: 204
Deux livres de chirurgie (A.P.): xvi, 141, 142, 208
Devils: 118

Diacalcitheos plaster: 137, 225
Dianne de France: 37, 58, 59, 157
Dionis, M*: 205
Dinners honoring Paré: 138, 139
Dionneau, Jacques*: 148, 167, 177
Disarmament of La Rochelle: 124
Discours de la Mumie, etc. (A.P.): xvii, 179, 185
Disguise
 at Doullens: 92
 at Hesdin: 81
Dislocations: 115, 141, 151
Dissections: 22, 39, 52, 57, 87, 166, 180
Distillations: 141
"Divine Drink": 99
Dix Livres de la Chirurgie, etc. (A.P.): xvi, 62, 113, 208
Doe, Janet: numerous citations
Dolet, Étienne, Publisher: xiii, 54, *218*
Donations by A.P: 55, 94, 96, 101, 126, 147, 162, 164, 189, 197
Doullens (Dourlan), France: 92
Dowry
 Jeanne Mazelin: 41
 Jeanne Paré: 96, 163
 Jacqueline Rousselet: 145
Drake, Sir Francis: xvii, xviii
Dressings: 79, 134
Dreux, battle of: xv, 108, 134
Drouet, Loys*: 41, 49, 216
DuBois, Guillaume*: 88, 162, 167
Ducci, Filippa: 37
Duchesse de Lorraine: 151
DuPrat, Antoine, Cardinal: 24, 40
DuPrat, Antoine, Provost of Paris: 188
DuPuy, Jacques (Printer): 174
DuPuytren, Musée: 203
Duret, Dr. Loys: 122, 148, 225
Dysentery, Epidemic: 92

E

Easter as New Year: 103, 117
Edict of Roussillon: 117
Edward VI, England: xiv
Egmont, Count: 93
Egyptiac: 137, 225
Eiffel Tower: 98

INDEX 239

d'Elbeuf, Count (Charles de Lorraine): 163, 227
Elbow, gunshot wound: 135
Elbow joint amputation: 34
Elizabeth, Austria: 140
　Queen, England: xv
　de Valois, Queen, Spain: xv, 121
Ellain, Dr.: 174
Embalming
　Charles IX: xvi, 148
　description of: 180
　François II: xv
　Henri III: 192
　M. de Martigues: 83
Emigration, religious: 142
Empirical medical care: 140
Emperor, Holy Roman Empire
　Charles V: 27, 75, 76, 89, *214*
　Ferdinand, Austria: 89
　Maximilian II: 140, *225*
Enchanter: 118
Enemas, milk, for dysentery: 92
d'Enghein, Duke (Jean de Bourbon): 67, *218*
Entertainment: 113, 116, 128, 138
d'Entragues, François de Balsac: 189, *228*
Epidemic
　dysentery, 92
　plague: xv, xvii, 45, 106, 110, 116, 133, 169
　smallpox, xv, 106, 126, 127
Epilepsy: 121
d'Eschevannes, C.: 118, 125, *223*
d'Estampes, Duke, Jean de Brosse: 45, 47, 79, *216*
　Duchesse, Anne de Pisseleu: 46, 58, 216, *229*
Estate, A.P.: 195
d'Este, Anne
　Duchesse de Guise: 95, *218*
　Duchesse de Nemours: 161, 196
Estienne, Dr. Charles: 41, 48, 51, *216*
l'Estoile, Pierre de, Journalist: 10, 193
l'Estrelle, M. Bernault de: 176, 180
d'Estres, M.: 68, 86
d'Eu, Count: 108
Eustace, M.*: 148
l'Evesque, wound: 35

Examinations
　College of Surgeons of St. Côme: 88
　Corporation of Barber-surgeons: 40
Excellence of Man (A.P.): 168
Execution
　by burning: 188
　for infanticide: 166
　Mary, Queen of Scots: 189
　Poltrot: 109
Expeditions (A.P.)
　Boulogne: xiii, 50, 55; Château-le-Comte: xv, 62; Court Tour: xvi, 111, 130; Dourlan: xv, 92; Dreux: xv, 108; Flanders: 136-140; Hesdin: xiv, 77-84; La Fère: xiv, 90; Landerneau: 46; Maroilles: 45; Metz: xiv, 61; Perpignan: xiii, 42; Plessis-les-Tours: xvi, 125; Rouen: xv, 104; Toul-Damvilliers: xiv, 61; Turin: xiii, 26, 28, 32
Experimentation
　antidote: 128
　criminals: 129
　potential cautery: 125
　surgery: 34
Eye
　"balm": 177
　diseases of: 174, 184, 187
　injury: 176
Ezelin, M. Nicole (Notary): 55

F

Faculté de Médecine: 21, 23, 40, 88, 131, 133, 153, 162, 165, 169, 174, 204, 205
Family
　litigation: 55, 188
　A. Paré: 195, 198
Famine, Paris: 193
de Farges (apothecary): 120
Farnese, Duke, Horace: 37, 68, 77, 80, *219*
de Felle, François: 95
Femur, gunshot wound: 89, 108, 136
Fencing injury: 176

Fernel, Dr. Jean: 19, 53, 88, 119, *213*
Fetus
  development: 141, 142
  malformation: 140
Fevers
  carbuncles: 122
  malaria: 92
  writing on: 168
le Fèvre (Lefèvre), Dr. Pierre: 105, 127, 148, 150, 171, *222*
Fire-arms, wounds by, etc. (Le Paulmier): 133
Fistula
  broncho-pleural: 36
  salivary, traumatic: 90
Five Books of Surgery (Paré): xvi, 101, 134, 141, 169
Flanders, trip to: 136-140
de Flexelles, Dr. Philippe: 52, *217*
Flight
  from plague: 170
  of Royal Family: 131
Florida, Huguenot colonization: xvi
de Foix, Claude, Duchesse de Laval: 13, *210*
la Fontaine, M. de, Chevalier: 122
Dr. Guy de: 180
Fontainebleau: xvi, 28, 112, 113
Fôrest, François: xvii, 165, 190, 192, 198
  François II: 192
  Jeanne Paré: 190, 192
le Fort, M.*: 183
Fournier, Charles: 56
Fractures: 141
  ankle (A.P.): xv, 98, 113
  leg: 68
  skull: 34, 69, 79, 106
Franco, Pierre*: 113, 223
François I, de Valois: xiii, 14, 24, 26, 39, 44, 52, 58, 103, 111, 201, *210*
François II, de Valois: xiii, xv, 94, 96
Frankfort, Germany: 132, 142
Fraudulent beggers: 53, 82, 100
French language: 18, 56
French Surgery (Dalechamps): 116
de Fronsac, Duke: 197

G

Gaignard, Dr. Robert: 88, 167
Galen, 54, 85, 154, 184, *212*
Garnier, Germain: 114
Garonne, river: 120
Garrison, F. H.: 187
Gascony, Gulf of: 123
Gaudin, Dr. Alexis: 148, 150, *225*
de Gaugier, Premier-Physician: 86
Gaultier:
  Claude: 126
  Dennis*: 189
  Jean: 126
Genealogy
  Paré: 11
  Valois-Bourbon: 12
Generation and *Monsters* (Paré): 154, 168
Generosity of Paré: 55, 94, 96, 101, 126, 127, 147, 162, 164, 189, 197
Geneva, Switzerland: 97
Germain, Marie: 114
Gifts to Paré: 47, 61, 68, 78, 86, 122, 135
Gilbert, M.*: 104
God parent
  Paré: 107, 165
  Paré children: 49, 56, 95, 96, 161, 162, 165, 169, 182
Godin, Nicolas: 22
Gohel, Jean, Inn Keeper: 183
de Goulaines, M.: 36
Gourmelen, Dr. Étienne, Dean: xvii, 50, 78, 129, 130, 153, 165, 170, 172, 186, *216*
Gout: 62, 66, 89, 141
le Grand, Dr.: 92
Grand Assembly of Notables: xvi, 127
Grand, Châlelet: 14
Grand children (A.P.): 189, 190, 193
Grangier, Dr. Dean: 182
Gravelines, France: 84, 85
Greaulme, Dr. Robert: 101
Greek terms: 101
Gualterot, Vivant (Publisher): 49
Guast, Captain: 92
Gueau, Guillaume: 101, 198
"Guidon" (Guy de Chauliac): 21, 119

INDEX

Guillemeau, Dr. Charles: 174
  Jacques*: xvii, 52, 103, 148, 149, 162, 167, 173, 182, 183, 187, 196, 203, *222*
Guise, France: 48
de Guise, Charles, Cardinal: 52, 94, 114, 190, *217*
  Claude (Duke d'Aumale): 52, 191, *217*
  François, Duke: xiii, xv, 50, 52, 60, 62, 65-76, 86, 91, 95, 104, 109, 114, 135, 161, *217*
  Henri, Duke: xv, xviii, 114, 135, 142, 161, 190, *224*
  Louis: Duke d'Aumale: 52
  Cardinal de Lorraine: 191, *217*
Gulf of Gascony: 123
Gunpowder
  Burns: 33
  Poisoning: 30, 33
Gunshot wounds: 30, 31, 33, 104, 133, 135
Gunshot wounds (A.P.): xiii, xiv, 48, 50, 52, 59, 62, 97, 113
Guy XVI, Duke de Laval: 11, 13, *210*, *216*
Guy XVII Claude, Duke de Laval: 13, 45, *210*
Guy de Chauliac: 17, 21, 119, 203, *212*
Guyenne, France: 123

H

Haberling, W.: 185
Habicot, Nocholas*: 204
Hamby, W. B.: numerous citations
Haultin, Dr. Jean: 165, 172, 174, 196, *227*
d'Havre (d'Auret), Marquis: 135, *224*
Head injuries: 34, 44
Head Injuries (A.P.): xv, 101, 144
Headache, arteriotomy: 122
Heart, wound of: 33
Hédelin
  Catherine Paré: 189
  Claude: 172, 196, 197
  François: 197
  Jacques: 197

Heinault: 45, 136, *216*
Hematuria: 42
Hemicrania: 122
Hemorrhage: 47, 62, 147
Hemostasis
  cautery: 62, 78, 170
  forceps: 178
  ligature: 62, 113, 130, 178
Hemothorax, traumatic: 47, *215*
Henri de Navarre (Henri IV): 77, 142, 148, 180, 191
Henri de Valois (Henri II): xiii, xiv, xv, 12, 27, 37, 44, 52, 59, 76, 93, 94, 103, 104, 156
  (Henri III): xvi, xvii, 12; Duke d'Anjou: 148; King of Poland: 148; Henri III: 148, 157, 190, 192, 211
Henry VIII (England): xiii, 26, 52
The Hermitage: 113
Heroïdes (Ovid): 197
Héron, Dr. Giles: 166, *227*
Heron, Mathurin*: 178
Herue, Pierre: 178
de Héry, Thierry: 25, 39, 51, 54, 64, 76, 97, 113, 176, *215*
Hesdin, France: xiv, 61, 63, 77-84, 85, 186
l'Heureux Accouchement des Femmes (Guillemeau): 174, 196
The "Highwayman": 192
Hippocras: 99
Hippocrates: 34, 151, 154, 178, *212*
de l'Hirondelle, rue: 40, 57, 194, 197
Honors (A.P.) in Heinault: 139
Hôpital St. Jacques Majori: 39
Horbeck, Giullis (Artist): 185
d'Hostel, Marie: 178
Hôtel-de-Ville: 109
Hôtel-de-St. Pierre: 143
Hôtel-Dieu, Paris: xiii, 14, 23, 24, 26, 36, 37, 39, 174, 203, *211*
Houllier, Dr. Jacques: 39, 100, *215*
Houses, A.P.: xv, 56, 57, 97, 145, 189, 194, 195, 198, 200
Hubert, Louis*: 167
  Richard*: 98, 108, 135, 167, *221*
de la Huchette, rue: 96

Huguenot: xv, 59, 96, 107, 124, 132, 144, 147, *221*
Humerus, bullet in: 105
Humor, A.P.: 186
Hunger in army: 60, 66
Hydatid mole: 150
Hysteria: 120, 125

I

Ile-de-la-Cité: 14, 199, *211*
Illiterate nobles: 90
Illustrations: 101, 141, 142, 156, 168
Imposters: 53, 82, 100, 118
Incantations: 119
Indians, American: 75
Infanticide: 166
Infections: 35, 91, 108, 110, 113, 134
Inquisition: 188
Insect Bites: 141
Instruments, surgical: 101, 178
Inventions: 101, 151, 152
Isaac Paré: xv, 95, 96

J

Jacquart, Dr.: 174
Jacqueline Paré: xvii, 169
Jacqueline Rousselet: xvi, xvii, 145, 161, 162, 163, 164, 169, 172, 174, 189, 195
Jarnac, France
  battle of, xvi
  Count de: 60
  court tour: 124
Jeanne Paré (niece): xvii, xviii, 96, 147, 156, 192
Jerusalem: 74
Johnson, Th.: viii, 176
Jordanus, Dr.: 182
Jouan, Abel: 111, 112, 121, 125
Joubert, Prof. Laurent: 119, 167
Jouin, H.: 229
Journeys in Divers Places (*Apologie*, A.P.): xvii, 28, 42, 46, 62, 171, 185, 209

K

Kellett, C. C.: 41
Keynes, G.: 29
King's touch: 121
Kings, Paré's Service to: 64, 155

L

La Charonne, Mme.: 196
La Fère: xiv, 90
La Fillé, Dr. Pierre: 183, 225
Lallement, Antoinette, 169; Estienne: 95; Jean, 169; Marie, 169
Lambert, Charles*: 79; Ishmael*: 167, 227; Nicole*: 54, 95, 120, 135, 148, *218*, *224*
Lamer, Dr. Pierre: 165, 227
Lance wound, deGuise: 50: Henri II: 93
Landerneau, France: xiii, 46
Landrecies, France: xiii, 45, 46, 48
Landsquenets: 60, 135, *218*
Langlois, Nicolaus*: 88, 162, 167, *219*
Languet, Hubert, Elector of Saxony: 142
Lansdale, M. H.: 201
La Rochelle, France: xvi, 124, 144
de Lassus, M.: vii, 198
da Laussac, Seigneur: 118
Laval, France: 10, 47, 205
  Duke de: Guy XVI: 11, 13, *210*, 216; Guy XVII: 13, 45, *210*
Lavernault, Nicole*: 44, 96, *221*
Law suits: 41, 51, 56, 95, 188
Lay surgical operators: 20
League, Catholic: xvii, 191
LeBrun, Louis*: 88, 167; Nicholas: 88
LeCharron, Marquise Thury: 185, 197
Le Comte, Dr.: 174
Le Fort, Raol*: 167; Rodolphe, 172, 177, *228*
Le Gay, Jean*: 70, 162, *220*
Le Grand, Noe: 203, 205, *220*
Le Gras, J.: 111
Le Havre, France: xvi, 110
Lent: 112

Le Paulmier, Dr. Julien: vii, 133, 141, 147, 223
Dr. Stephen: numerous citations
Le Rat, Captain: 6
Le Roy, Dr. Jacques: 127
Libraries, Bibliothèque Nationale: 111, 165; St. Genevieve, 161
Licenses, Paré
  Master Barber-Surgeon: xiii, 25, 40
  Sworn-Surgeon: xiv, 88
Liebault, Dr. Jean: 165, 178, 227
Ligature in amputations: xvi, 62, 130, 133
Lille, Belgium: 63
Artificial limbs: 59, 62
Lind, L. R.: 213
Lithotomy, bladder: 146; salivary duct: 122
Loan: 56
Loire river: 124, 191
Loquet, Guillaume: 165
de L'Orme, Philibert, Architect: 152
de Lorraine,
  Charles, Cardinal: 58, 94, 190, 191
  Charles-le-Grand, Duke: 14
  Marquis d'Elbeuf: 163, 227
  Duchesse, Claude de Valois: xvii, 114, 151
  François (see deGuise)
Louis XI (Saint Louis): 24, 27, 214
  XIII: 174
  XIV: 58, 131
  XV: 58
  XVI: 58
Louvre: 14, 87, 143
de Lude, Court: 68
Lung, gunshot wound: 80
Lusson, Dr. Guillaume: 165
Luxembourg: 48, 61
Lying, accusation: 151
Lyon, France: 28, 42
  Archbishop: xviii, 191, 228
  Plague (1564): 116

M

Mâcon, France: 116

Magic: 155; in therapy: 82
de Magnane, M.: 68
Maison de Trois Maures (3 Moors): xv, 56, 97, 194, 200
  de la Vache: 56, 97, 145, 195, 198
Maisons de pesta (pest houses): 170
Malaria: 92
Maleziev, Andre*: 166, 227
Malformations, congenital: 95
Malgaigne, J. F.: numerous citations
Malta, siege of: 125
de Mamères, Anne and Estienne: 182
Mammary gland; blood supply: 167
de Mansfield, Count Charles: 163, 227;
  Count Pierre-Ernest, 134, 224
Manuscripts, translations: 16
Maps
  Court tour: 112
  Expeditions to Maroilles and Landerneau: 46; Metz-Hesdin: 61; Perpignan: 43; Turin: 28
  Paré neighborhood: 199, 202
  Paris, 16th century: 15
Marc, Nicolas*: 177
Marcel, Étienne: 14
Marchant, Jacques*: 196, 229
la Mare, Mlle: 117
Maréschal, M. Jacques: 182
Marescot, Dr. Michel: 165
Margot, Queen: see Marguerite de Valois
Marguerite de Valois: 1, 77, 93, 127, 142
Marie Paré: xvii, 164
Marie Stuart, Queen of Scots: xv, xviii, 94, 96, 189, 221
Maroilles, expedition to: xiii, 45; map: 46
de Marque, Jacques*: 204
Marriage Contract: A.P.-J. Mazelin: 41, A.P.-J. Rousselet: 145; J. Paré-Viart: 163; J. Paré-Fôrest: 190
Marseilles, France: 119
de Martigues, Vicount, Charles de Luxembourg: 68, 77, 83, 219
Martin, Catherine Paré: 11, 14; Didier: 172; Gaspard: 11, 14, 96, 130

Martin, Dr. Jean: 166, 227
Mary Stuart, Queen of Scots: see Marie-
Mary Tudor: xiv, xv
Massacre, St. Bartholomew's Day, xvi, 142; Vassy: xv
Mathurins, church of: 88
Maubert, Place: 93, *218*
Maureval, M: 143
Mauriceau, M.°: 205
Maurois, André: *213, 221*
Maximillian II, Emperor: 140, *225*
de Mayenne, Duke: 193
Mayenne, river: 13
Mazelin, Jean: 24
    Jeanne: xiii, xvi, 24, 40, 41, 49, 95, 96, 145, 195, 198
Mazille, Dr. Jean: 118, 144, 147, 148, *223*
Median nerve injury: xvi, 127
Medical heirarchy, 16th century: 18
    illustration
    scene, Paris, 16th century: 18
    school, Paris: 203
    superstitions: 181
de' Médicis, Catherine: ix, xiii, xv, 18, 52, 77, 104, 118, 152, 191, *212*
Memory, A. P.: 85
de Mendoce, Duke: 103
Menegaux, G.: 26
Mestreau, Jean: 56, 97, 200
Méthode curatoire de la Maladie vénérienne (de Héry): 64
La Methode curative des playes, et fractures de la teste humain, etc. (A.P.): xv, 102, 207
La méthode de traicter les playes faictes par hacquebutes, etc. (A.P.): xiii, 48, 59, 207
Metz, France: map: 61; A.P. trip: xiv, 61; siege: 62, 66-76, 187
Meudon, France: A.P.: 57, 58, 192; archer of: 146
Midwife: 196
Miereveldt, Artist: 185
Mignon, Jean: 55
Milan physician: 37
Military intelligence: 85

medicine: 27
surgery: 30
Milk, for dysentery: 92
Millet, Dr.: 88
Miron, Dr. Marc: 151, 174, *226*
Mistress, of Charles IX: 125; François I: 46, 58, 216, *229;* Henri II: 37, 58, 59, 157
Moliere, Jean Baptiste: 58
Mombeau, Christophle°: 150
de Monantheuil, Dr. Henri: 161, 169, 173, *226*
Moncontour, battle of: xvi, 134
Monseigneur (François de Valois, duke d'Anjou): xvii, 114, 134
Monsters: 140, 141
Monsters and Prodigies (A.P.): 95, 123
Mont Cenis: 3
Montaigne, Michel: 19, 115
Mont-de-Marsan, 123
de Montejan, René, Duke: xiii, 4, 27, 32, 37, 113, *214*
de Montespedon, Phillipes: 33, 163, 164, *215*
de Montgomery, Gabriel, Duke: xv, 93, 104, *221*
Montmartre: 58, 100
de Montmorency, Anne, Constable: 13, 27, 52, 59, 86, 89, 94, 95, 108, 112, 113, 118, 124, 132, 134, *214*
    Anne (Duchesse de Laval): 13, 171
    Duchesse: 132
    François: 68, 77
    Henri (Marshal): 134
Montpellier, France: xvi, 119
de Montpensier, Louis de Bourbon, Duke: 67, 114, *218*
    Princesse: 183
de Montruil, Pierre, Architect: 103
Mortality, battle wound: 91, 108, 110, 134
Moses: 119
Motto, Paré
    "Fin est la mort - - -": 133
    "Je le pensay - - - - -": 7
    "Labor improbus - - -": 98, 101, 168
Moulins, Grand Assembly: xvi, 127
de Mouron, Dr.: 172
Moussey, M. Vincent, Councillor: 172

INDEX

Moynihan, Lord Berkeley: 185
Mummy, as drug: 172, 177
Mumy, Discours de la, etc. (A.P.): xvii, 179, 185
Musée, Carnivalet: 201; Dupuytren: 203
Museum, A.P.: 57, 123, 140; Carnivalet, 201; Dupuytren, 203; Mevdon: 58
Mythologic monsters: 141

N

Nancy, France: xiv, xvii, 61, 151
Napoleon: vii, 198
Naquier, Jean: 55
Naval attack: 46
de Navarre, Duke, King,
  Antoine de Bourbon: xv, 94, 98
  Henri de Bourbon: xv, 114, 142, 144, 148, 192
Neighborhood, Paré, map: 199
Nemours, France: 197
de Nemours, Jacques de Savoy, Duke: 95, 196, *218*
Nerve injury, Charles IX, xvi, 127, 148
Nesnager, Nicholas: 183
Nestle, tower: 14, *211*
Nestor, Dr. Jean: 98, *221*
de Neufville, Marie Paré: 96
des Nuex, François*: 88, 167: Nicole Rasse*: 167, *220*
de Nevers, François de Cleves, Duke: 89, *220*
New Year: xvi, 102, 103, 117, *214*
Nose bleed: 122
Nostradamus, Dr. Michel: 118, *223*
Notables, Grand Assembly of: 127
Nôtre-Dame Cathedral: 14, 24, *211*
la Noue, Jerome de: 167, *228*

O

Occult: 118
Odes (Ronsard): 56
d'Odet, Marshal: 13
Les Oeuvres de M. Ambroise Paré:
xvii, 29, 33, 52, 98, 113, 152, 153, 155, 156, 163, 165, 168, 171, 173, 175, 179, 184, 190, 205, 208, 209
Oil burns: 33; of puppies: 32
Onion poultices for burns: 33
l'Opera Ambroisii Parei, etc.: xvii, 163, 173, 175, 209
Ophthalmology, 188
d'Orange, Prince: 93
Orbit, injury: 176
d'Orléans, Duke, Henri de Valois: 114
Orléans, France: 108, 125, 189
Orthopedic appliances: 59, 109
Osteomyelitis, ankle: 178; femur: 136; skull: 36
Ovid: 197
Oxycrate: 127, 177, *228*

P

Packard, F. P., vii, 115
Paget, Stephen: vii, 21, 51, 57, 88, 162, 163, 172, 173
Painting, oil, of A.P.: 185, 197
Palace, Chaillot: 98
Palais d'Amour: *229*
de Paley, Chateau: 149, *229*
Palissy, Bernard, Ceramist: 152, *226*
Paper making: 17
Paracelsus: 170, 203, *228*
Paradis, Louis*: 176
Paraphimosis: 37
Paraplegia: 132, 177
Paré, Ambroise: birth: xiii, 10, 12; parents: 11; genealogy: 11; siblings: 11; age: 210; youth: 13; education: 36, 54; apprenticeship: 14, 23, 42: to Paris: 13; at Hôtel-Dieu: 25, 26; military service: 26, 27; to Turin: 26-28, 32; discovery re gunshot wounds: 31; garrison life: 32-47; poetry: 36; admission to Corp. Barber-surgeons: 25, 40; marriage, Jeanne Mazelin: 40-41; to Pergignan: 42; Maroilles: 46; Landerneau: 46; Landrecies: 45-48; first book, *Gunshot wounds*: 48; first child, François: 48-49;

Briefve Collection (anatomy): 48; houses: 56, 57; appointment Surgeon-in-Ordinary: 64; to Metz: 61, 67-76; capture at Hesdin: 81; admission to College of Surgeons: 88; to La Fère: 90; Doullens: 92; Death Henri II: 94; 2nd child, Isaac: 95, 96; 3rd child, Catherine: 96; Death François II: 96, move to Trois Maures: 97; *Anatomie universelle*: 97, 101, 207: fracture ankle: 98, 113; book of *Head Injuries*: 102; appointment, Premier-Surgeon: 103, 149; to Bourges: 104; Rouen: 104; poisoning: 106; religious status: 106; to Dreux: 108; Le Havre: 110; Court tour: 111-130; *Ten Books of Surgery*: 113; operation on Gaspard Martin: 130; Book on *The Plague*, etc.: 132; trip to Flanders: 136; *Five Books of Surgery*: 141; *Two Books of Surgery*: 142; St. Bartholomew's Day Massacre: 142; death Jeanne Mazelin Paré: 145; remarriage, Jacqueline Rousselet: 145; autopsy, Charles IX: 148; appointment Premier-Surgeon to Henri III: 149; trip to Nancy: 115; *Les Oeuvres*: 153; birth 4th child, Anne: 161; birth 5th child, Ambroise (II): 162; death Ambroise (II): 163; birth 6th child, Marie: 164; A.P. godfather: 165; *Les Oeuvres*, ed. 2: 166, 168; birth 7th child, Jacqueline: 169; book on *Plague*, etc.: 170; birth 8th child, Catherine: 172; l'Opera (ed. 3 of *Oeuvres*): 173, 175; marriage Catherine (I) Paré to F. Mazelin: 173; book on *Mummy, Unicorn* and *Plague*: 179; birth and death of last, 9th, child, Ambroise III: 183; *Les Oeuvres*, ed. 4, with *Apologie*, etc.: 184-187; laws vs. F. Mazelin: 188, recording of his will: 189; birth grand-daughter: 190; second grandchild: 190; meeting with Archbishop de Lyon: 194; death of A.P.: 194; The Paré Family: 195-198; his property: 198-203; surgical influence: 203-206; statue in Laval: 205; books: 207-209

Paré, Ambroise II, 5th child: 162, 163
Ambroise III, 9th child: xvii, 183, 184
Anne, 4th child, baptism: 161; delivery: 174; marriage Henri Simon: 189, 195
Bertrand, nephew: 54
Catherine I, 3rd child: xv, xvii, 96, 172; marriage F. Rousselet: 173; 190
Catherine II, 8th child: xvii, 172; marriage François Hédelin: 197
Catherine Paré Martin, Sister: 96, 130
François, first child: xiii, 49
Isaac, 2nd child: xv, 95, 96
Jacqueline, 7th child: xvii, 169
Jean, Barber-surgeon, brother: 11, 13, 54
Jean, Trunk-maker, brother: 11, 14, 55, 96, 198
Jeanne, niece: xvii, xviii, 96, 147, 163, 178, 183, 190, 192
Marie, 6th child: xvii, 164
Paré property: 189
Parents, A.P.: 11
Paris, of 16th century: 14; siege: xviii, 192
16th century map: 15; medical scene: 16
Parlement: 18, 41, 165, *212*
Parvis Notre-Dame: 24
Patin, Dr. Guy: 174
Payment, medical attendants: 151; A.P.: 76, 86, 151
Peace, of Amboise: xvi, 109; Château-Cambriesis: 93
Pelvic synostoses: 167
Perier, Barbe: 55; Catherine: 55; Claude: 101, 198; François: 55, 101, 198; Marie: 14, 55, 101
Perpignan expedition: xiii, 42

INDEX

Pest-houses: 170
Peyrilhe, M., 88
Philip II, Spain: xv, 89, 93, 191, 220
Philippe-Auguste: 14
Philippe-le-Bel: 22
(Phlebotomy) Bleeding: 99; Charles IX: 127; for plague: 117, for smallpox: 127
Picardy: 45, 76, 77, 92
Picart, Nicolas°: xvii, 115, 151
de Pichonnat, Francois: 147, 198
de Pienne, M: 69
Piètre, Dr. Simon: 144, 148, 167, 174, 177, 225
Pigeon-blood balm: 177
Pigray, Pierre°: xviii, 108, 134, 167, 171, 177, 191, 192, 203, 222 224
Pineau, Dr. Severin: 116, 167, 203 227
Pirating publication: 48
de Pisseleau, Anne, Countess d'Estampes: 46, 58, 216
Place-de-Grève: 109
Place Maubert: 93, 218
  St. André-des-Arts: 201
  St. Michel: 200, 201
  de Vosges: 93
Plagiarism: 48, 52, 133, 182
Plague, Council: 169; Le Havre: 110; Lyon (1564): 116; Paré attack: 133; Paris (1562); xv, 106, 172 (1580): xvii, 169; Perpignan: 45
The Plague, etc. (A.P.): xvi, xvii, 133, 170, 182
Pléiade: 56
Plessis-les-Tours, France: xvi, 125, 134, 191
Pleuro-bronchial fistula: 36
Podalic version: 54
Poetry: 56, 159, A.P.: 36, 56, 159, 173, 188
Poisoning, accusation: 96, 162; of A.P.: xv, 106; thief: 129; of wounds: 105, 110
de Poitiers, Dianne: 37, 59, 95, 201
Poltrot, Jean, assassin: 109
Ponce de Leon: xiii
du Pont, M: 78
Pont St. Michel: 57, 163, 193

Pope: 191; Clement VII: 154
Poullet, Daniel°: xvii, 183
Portail, Antoine: xvi, xviii, 92, 98, 127, 134, 148, 149, 167, 191, 192, 203, 220
Porte d' Auteil: 132
Portraits, A.P.: 97, 101, 141, 142, 159, 168, 179, 185
Posson, Toussant: 183
Potential cautery: 121, 125
Poullet, Daniel°: 183
Power, Dr. D'Arcy: 185
Premier Barber-Surgeon: 23, 131
Premier-Physicians: de Bourges: 53; Chapelain; 118, de Gaugier: 86; Mazille: 118, 144; deSalon: 95
Premier-Surgeons: Lavernault: 44, 96; Paré xv, xvii, 103, 149, 190
de Prime, Catherine: 56; Jacqueline: 92; Jeanne: 41, 49, 96; Loys: 96; Méry: 40, 56, 147, 198; Odo: 41
Printing, impact of: 17
Prohibited books: 97
Property, A.P.: 198, 203; map: 199
Prostheses: 36, 59, 62, 109
Provence: xvi, 118
Publishers: Jean de Brie: 59, 97; Buon: 149, 166, 170, 184; Cavellat: 53; Colines: 48, 51; Dolet: xiii, 54, 218; DuPuy: 174; Gualterot: 49, 54; Roelants: 52; Rondel: 149, 190; le Royer: 97 Sucevin: 59, 97; Wechel: 132, 141, 142, 149

R

Rabelais, François: 19, 59
de Randan, M: 68
Ransom: 81
Ranula: 122
Rasse, François°: 62
Rebellion, religious: 124
Rebors, Dr. Claude: 166, 174, 227
Rebuttal: 134, 141, 142
Record, M.: 60
Regency, Charles IX: 97, 109, 147; François I: 94
Regulation of surgeons: 22

Reims, France: 52, 64, 100
Religion, A.P.: 106; Wars of: xv, xvi, xviii, 104, 131, 144
Renaissance, spread to France: 10
Renaud, Antoine°: 183
Renouart, Captain: 35
Replique . . . a la Response faicte contre son Discours de la Licorne, A.P.: 182, 209
Reproduction, human: 141
Response: Le Paulmier to Paré: 142; Paré to Gourmelen: 153; Paré, re: Unicorn horn: 183
de Retz, Count: 113, 118, 147, 192
Richelieu, Cardinal: 197
Ridicule of medical superstitions: 181
Rigault, Dr.: 96
Ringrave, de Daun, Count Jean Philippe II: 60, 113, 135, *218*
Riolan, Dr. Jean: 89, 144, *220*
Risch-Leon: 189
River, Canche: 78; Garonne: 120; Loire: 124; Mayenne: 13; Sâone: 116; Seine: 14, 98, 130
Rivière, Étienne de la: 41, 48, 62, 87, 99, 103, 134, *215*
Robbery during plague: 117
de Rochefoucould, M.: 68
de Rochelle, Marquis: 202
la Roche-sur-yon, Prince de, Charles de Bourbon: 67, 94, 105, 114, 122, 124, 218
  Princesse, Philippes de Montespedon: 33, 163, 164, *215*
Roelants, Jan, Publisher: 52
Roger, madame: 149
de Rohan, François: 95
  Vicount, René: xiii, xiv, 42, 45, 49, 50, 53, 55, 59, 60, 62, 95
Rome, sack of: xiii
Rondel, Jeanne, Publisher: 149, 190; Nicholas: 149
Rondelet, M: 123
de Ronsard, Pierre, poet: 19, 56, 159, *213*
Rotisserie Perigourdine: 201
Rouen, France: xv, 104, 105, 113, 134, 193
Rousselet, Antoine: 24; Barbe: 172; Catherine Paré: 145, 190; Charles: 193; Dr. Claude: 165; Florentine: 190; François: xvii, 173, 188, 190, 195; Jacqueline: xvi, xvii, 145, 161, 162, 163, 164, 172, 174, 189, 195; Jacques: 145, 165; Nicholas: 190
Rousset, François°: 173
Roussillon, Château: xvi, 117; Edict of: xvi, 117
le Roy, Dr. Jacques: 113, *223*
Royal College of Surgeons, England: 185
de Roye, Marquis: 81
le Royer, Jean, Engraver & Publisher: 97, 113
Rue, des Augustins: 198; Battoire, 202; Bethisy: 143; de la Boucherie: 203; des Cordeliers: 203; de l'École de Médicine: 203; Garanciere: 189; Gît-le-Coeur: 202; de la Harpe: 203; Hautefeville: 203; de l'Hirondelle: 40, 57, 194, 198; de l'Huchette: 96; des Pretres-St. Severin: 146; Prouvaires, 195; St. André-des-Arts: 40, 41, 200; St. Denis: 177; St. Honoré: 183; St. Jacques: 101, 102-146; St. Severin: 203; des Verbois: 178
la Rue, Pierre de, tailor: 56, 163

S

Sacre-Coeur: 58
Saillard, Dr. Antoine: 39
Saint
  de St. André, Jacques d'Albon, Count: 52, 60, 67, *217*
  St. André-des-Arts, church: xviii, 41, 95, 96, 106, 145, 161, 163, 164, 165, 169, 172, 182, 194, 200; rue: 40, 41, 200
  St. Aubin, Captain: 92
  St. Bartholomew's Day Massacre: xvi, 142
  Sainte-Châpelle: 103
  St. Cloud: 192

INDEX

St. Côme, College of Surgeons of: 23, 44, 88, 153, 162, 174, 203; Confraternity of: 22, 23, 88, 131
Sts. Cosmo and Damien: 21
St. Denis, France: 63, 134; battle: xvi, 131; rue: 177
St. Genevieve, Library: 161
de St. Germain, Jean, Apothecary: 55
St. Germain l'Auxerrois: 143
St. Germain-des-Fosses: 128
St. Germain-des-Pres: 50, 189
St. Germain-en-Laye: 77, 103, 147
St. Germain-le-Viele: 197
St. Innocents', cemetery: 229; church: 134
St. Jacques-de-la-Boucherie, church: 88
St. Jacques, rue: 101, 102, 146
St. Jean d'Angely: 124
St. Jean-de-Luz: 122
de St. Jean-en-Dauphine, M.: 68
St. Just: 127
St. Landry, Bishop: 24
St. Louis (Louis XI): 24, 27, 102, *214*
St. Martin of the Fields: 178
St. Michel, bridge: 57, 163, 193; Place: 40, 42, 57, 200, 201
St. Nicholas, France: xiv, 62
St. Omer, France: 85
de St. Pont, M.°: 148, *225*
de St. Pris, M.: 118
St. Quentin, battle: xiv, 89
St. Sepulcre, church: 21, 40
St. Severin, church: 146; rue: 203
Salamander, 201
Salerno, School of: 16
Salivary, duct stones: 122; fistula: 90
Salon, France: 118
de Salon, Dr. Joachim: 95
Salt tax: 94
Sambuc (elders), oil of: 30
de Sancerre, Count: 60
de Santerre, Mme: 196
Sâone, river: 116
Sarcasm, A.P.: 66, 78

Satire, A.P.: 66, 78
Saul, King: 119
de Saulx, Gaspard: 116
Saumur, France: 125, 191
de Savoy
   Charles-Emmanuel, Duke de Nemours: 161, *219*
   Jacques, Duke de Nemours: 95, 161, *218*
   Philippe, Duke: xv, 77, 89, 93, 161, *218, 219*
Saxony, Elector of: 142
Scalp avulsion: 79
Scrofula: 121
Secret, cautery: 126; wound "balm": 32
Sedan, France: 61
Segregation of patients: 170
Seguier, Criminal-Lieutenant: 180
Seguier, Pierre, Chevalier: 165
Seine, river: 14, 98, 130
Senlis, France: 171
Sens, France: 114, 130
Sequestra: 137
Sex, change of: 115
Sezanne, France: 94
Sheepskin dressing: 177
Shoulder, dislocations: 151; gunshot wound: 104, 135
Side-saddle: 114
Siege of, Château-le-Comte: 63; Hesdin: xiv, 77-86, La Rochelle, 144; Le Havre: 110; Malta: 125; Metz: xiv, 66-76; Paris: xviii, 192; Perpignan: xiii, 42; Rouen: xv, 104, 105, 113, 134, 193; Theroüenne: xiv, 77, 85
Simon, Anne Paré: 174, 189, 195; Henri: 195, 196
Singer, D. W.: 41
Siret, M.°: 134
Skull, injuries: 34, 36, 69, 79, 106
Smallpox: xv, xvi, 106, 126, 127
Snake bite: xvi, 120, 127
Spanish, Armada: xviii, soldiers, cruelty of: 75, 81
Spine, injuries: 132, 177
Spirits: 119

250   AMBROISE PARÉ

Spy: 90
States-General, Blois: xviii, 190
Statue, A.P.: 205
Statutes, College of St. Côme: 162
Street plan, Paré area: 199, 202
Stuart, Marie, Queen of Scots: xv, xviii, 94, 96, 189, *221*
Sucevin, Agnes, publisher: 59, 97
Sunstroke: 123
Superstition, medical: 181
Surgeon-in-Ordinary: xiv, xv, 64, 94, 97
Surgeons, Master: 22; regulation: 22; St. Côme: 204; Sworn (to the Châtelet): 22, 205; Wandering: 20
Surgery, development in Paris: 20; Military: 30; 16th Century: 19
Surgical influence of A.P.: 203-206
Suza, Pass: 3; battle of: 29
Sylvius (Jacques duBois): xiii, xiv, 24, 39, 49, 54, 89, *215*
Sworn-Surgeons: 22, 205
Syphilis: 39, 52

T

Tables Anatomiques (Guillemeau): 173
de la Taste: Dr.: 120
Ten Books of *Surgery* (A.P.): xvi, 62, 113, 208
Tendon injury: 108
Terrasse, The: 58
Têt, river: 42
Tetanus: 35
Theriac: 30, 119, *214*
Therouënne: 77, 85
Thiboutot, M.: 189
Thief: 117, 128
Thigh, gunshot wounds: 30, 33, 136
Thionville, France: 62, 75
Thorax, gunshot wound: 80, sword wound: 35
de Tillet, Anne: 95; Maric: 165; Seraphin: 95
Titus, Emperor: 74

Torino, Italy: xiii, 3, 27, 28
Torture, of captives: 81; of Poltrot: 109
Touchet, Marie: 125, 140, 189, *223*
Toul, France: xiv, 61
de la Tour d'Auvergne, Madelaine: 128
Tour de Nestle: 14, *211*
Tour du Coin: 14
Tournai, Belgium: 63
Tournament: 93, 128
Tournelles Castle: 14, 87, 93, 152
Tours, France: 134, 140
Traicté . . . playes de pistole, etc. (Le Paulmier): 133
Traicté de la peste, etc. (A.P.): xvi, xvii, 133, 170, 182, 208
Traite des maladies de l'oeuil (Guillemeau): 187
Traitté . . . Enfantement Caesarien (Rousset): 173
Treatise on Arquebusades (Joubert): 119
Treaty of Vancelles: 77
Trepan: 69, 106
Trial, legal: 95, 155, 188
de la Trosse, M.: 128
de Troyes, Jean°: 146
Tuilerie Palace: 152
Tumor, examination of: 150
Turin, Italy: xiii, 3, 27, 28
Turner, E.: 11, 200, 229
Twins, Duchesse de Lorraine: 150; fetus: 140
Two Books of Surgery (A.P.): xvi, 141, 142

U

Ulcer, decubitus: 136; painful: 183; varicose: 84
Unicorn horn: 180, 182
Universities, development: 16
Uremia: 132
Urology: 113
de Ursins, M. Christophe Jouvenel: xvii, 68, 178, 179, *228*
Uterus, dissection: 149, 150
d' Usés, Duke: 142, 178

INDEX

V

Valet-de-chambre, A.P.: xv, xvii, 95, 149
Valet, Paul: 165, 183, 222
Vallée, Alexander: 185, 228
de Valois, Catherine (Queen Spain): 93; Claude, Duchesse de Lorraine: 114, 151; François, Duke d'Anjou, Monseigneur: 114-134; Herculé, Duke d'Alençon: 106; Henri, Duke d'Orléans, 114, 192; King of Poland: 148, King, Henri III: 148; Marguerite (I): 1, 77, 93, 127; Marguerite (II): 142
Valois-Bourbon Genealogy: 12
Valsalva maneuver: 36
Varicose ulcer: 84
Vassy, "massacre": xv
Vaterre, Dr. Michel: 148, 225
Vaucelles, Treaty of: 77
de Vaudeveille, M.: 14, 84, 85
"Velvet" cautery: 126
de Vendôme, Antoine de Bourbon, Duke: 63, 64, 217; François: 68, 219
Venereal Diseases (de Héry): 64
of Venins (A.P.): 169
Verdun, trip to: xiv, 61
Vernacular writing: 155, 160
Versailles, France: 59
Version, podalic: 54
Vesalius (André Vésale): xii, xv, 24, 40, 48, 84, 93, 101, 213
Vespasian, Emperor: 74
le Vest, Barnabe*: 88, 219
Viart, Ambroise: xvii, 165; Claude: xvii, 156, 163, 165, 167, 173, 177, 178, 183, 198, 226; Jeanne Paré: xvii, xviii, 163, 165, 183, 190
de Vigny, François: 183

de Vigo, Jean: 7, 21, 30, 40, 203, *213*
Vigor, Dr. Regnault: 148, 151, *225*
de Villars, Marquis: 77
Villaume, M.: 197
Ville-du-Bois, France: 189, 196
de Villenueve, Dr. François: 49
de Villeville, Marshal: 67, *219*
Vimont, Dr.: 205
de Violanes, Dr. Oliver: 150, *225*
Vipers: 120, 127
Vitré, France: 27

W

Wandering surgeons: 20
War, "of The 3 Henris": xviii; of Religion: xv, xvi, xviii, 104, 131, 144
Wechel, Publisher, André: 132, 141, 142, 149; Christian: 132
Wedding presents: 163
Whaling at Biarritz: xvi, 123
Wilhelm, M. Jacques: 201
Will, of A.P.: xviii, 189
Williams, H. N.: 37
Wine, Burgundy: 116
Witchcraft: xviii, 118, 120, 188
Witness: 41, 95, 145, 148, 151
The Works (A.P.): xvii, xviii, 29, 33, 52, 98, 113, 152, 153, 155, 156, 163, 171, 173, 175, 179, 184, 190, 205, 208-209
Wounds, gunshot: 30, 31, 33, 104, 133, 135; heart: 33; nerves: 141; Thorax: 35, 80
Wrestling injury: 47

Y

Ynard, M*: 88
Youth of A.P.: 13